Register Now for Online Access to Your Book!

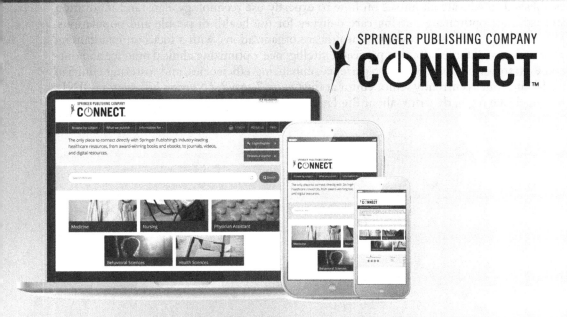

SPRINGER PUBLISHING COMPANY

CONNECT™

Your print purchase of *Emerging Technologies for Nurses* **includes online access to the contents of your book**—increasing accessibility, portability, and searchability!

Access today at:

http://connect.springerpub.com/content/book/978-0-8261-4651-9 or scan the QR code at the right with your smartphone and enter the access code below.

T2BN4PP6

Scan here for quick access.

SPRINGER / PUBLISHING COMPANY

View all our products at springerpub.com

Whende M. Carroll, MSN, RN-BC, is an informatics specialist with over 20 years of experience in nursing, as well as the dynamic universe of health information technology. As a nurse technologist, Whende has founded Nurse Evolution, a cause-based nursing community established to educate all nurses on how to expertly use technology, data, and innovation strategies for optimizing nursing care delivery for the health of people and populations. Whende has served as an advisor to healthcare organizations, with a focus on maintaining the nursing workforce, adopting precision intelligence, optimizing clinical practice and outcomes, transforming the patient experience, enhancing efficiencies, and fostering clinician well-being. She is currently senior editor at the *Online Journal of Nursing Informatics* (OJNI), for which she regularly writes about Big Data-enabled emerging technologies.

Emerging Technologies for Nurses

Implications for Practice

Whende M. Carroll, MSN, RN-BC

Editor

SPRINGER PUBLISHING COMPANY

First Springer Publishing edition 2021
No part of this publication may be reproduced, stored in a retrieval system, or transmitted in any form or by any means, electronic, mechanical, photocopying, recording, or otherwise, without the prior permission of Springer Publishing Company, LLC, or authorization through payment of the appropriate fees to the Copyright Clearance Center, Inc., 222 Rosewood Drive, Danvers, MA 01923, 978-750-8400, fax 978-646-8600, info@copyright.com or on the Web at www.copyright.com.

Springer Publishing Company, LLC
11 West 42nd Street
New York, NY 10036
www.springerpub.com
http://connect.springerpub.com

Acquisitions Editor: Joseph Morita
Compositor: S4Carlisle Publishing Services

ISBN: 978-0-8261-4649-6
ebook ISBN: 978-0-8261-4651-9
DOI: 10.1891/9780826146519

Instructor's Materials: Qualified instructors may request supplements by emailing textbook@springerpub.com:
Instructor's Manual ISBN: 978-0-8261-5197-1
Instructor's PowerPoints ISBN: 978-0-8261-5198-8

20 21 22 23 / 5 4 3 2 1

The author and the publisher of this Work have made every effort to use sources believed to be reliable to provide information that is accurate and compatible with the standards generally accepted at the time of publication. Because medical science is continually advancing, our knowledge base continues to expand. Therefore, as new information becomes available, changes in procedures become necessary. We recommend that the reader always consult current research and specific institutional policies before performing any clinical procedure. The author and publisher shall not be liable for any special, consequential, or exemplary damages resulting, in whole or in part, from the readers' use of, or reliance on, the information contained in this book. The publisher has no responsibility for the persistence or accuracy of URLs for external or third-party Internet websites referred to in this publication and does not guarantee that any content on such websites is, or will remain, accurate or appropriate.

Library of Congress Cataloging-in-Publication Data

Names: Carroll, Whende M., editor.
Title: Emerging technologies for nurses : implications for practice /
    Whende M. Carroll, editor.
Description: First Springer Publishing edition. | New York : Springer
    Publishing Company, 2021. | Includes bibliographical references and
    index.
Identifiers: LCCN 2019056412 (print) | LCCN 2019056413 (ebook) | ISBN
    9780826146496 (paperback) | ISBN 9780826146519 (ebook)
Subjects: MESH: Nursing Informatics | Data Science | Nursing--trends
Classification: LCC RT50.5 (print) | LCC RT50.5 (ebook) | NLM WY 26.5 |
    DDC 610.730285--dc23
LC record available at https://lccn.loc.gov/2019056412
LC ebook record available at https://lccn.loc.gov/2019056413

Contact us to receive discount rates on bulk purchases.
We can also customize our books to meet your needs.
For more information please contact: sales@springerpub.com

Whende M. Carroll: https://orcid.org/0000-0002-1062-6029

Printed in the United States of America.

To Catherine, George, Ian, and Jason

—with gratitude and joy.

Contents

Contributors

Whende M. Carroll, MSN, RN-BC Founder, Nurse Evolution, Senior Editor, *Online Journal of Nursing Informatics* (OJNI), University Place, Washington

Thomas R. Clancy, MBA, PhD, RN, FAAN Clinical Professor Ad Honorem, University of Minnesota School of Nursing, Minneapolis, Minnesota

Barbara Ficarra, RN, BSN, MPA Health Care Consultant, Health Educator, Multimedia Host, Barbara Ficarra Productions, LLC, Founder, Healthin30.com, Administrative Supervisor (Clinical and Patient Care), Hackensack Meridian Health, Hackensack University Medical Center, Hackensack, New Jersey

Kathleen A. McCormick, PhD, RN, FAAN, FACMI, FHIMSS Principal/ Owner, SciMind, LLC, North Potomac, Maryland

Foreword

It seems more apparent each day that technology is shaping our lives in new and impactful ways. Whether in our homes, offices, classrooms, or labs, we are increasingly reliant on technology to help us work faster, smarter, and better. So, as nurses, it is no surprise that emerging technologies are rapidly influencing healthcare and will soon dramatically change our practice. We must prepare ourselves to embrace innovation while we carefully consider the implications for transforming care delivery. As new technologies are adopted, nurses must be vigilant in monitoring quality and ensuring patient safety across the continuum of care. All the more reason to embrace this book as a vehicle to learn and prepare for the inevitable transformation. I hope that you are ready for the challenge because this resource will take you on a virtual journey to the future of nursing.

Nurses are natural innovators. *Emerging Technologies for Nurses: Implications for Practice* reminds us that we also have a responsibility to use evidence to make sure that the use of technology is combined with clinical understanding so that workflow is enabled and care is not compromised. Nurses are the optimal stakeholders to influence and inform the application of technology in healthcare. Now that we have near ubiquitous adoption of electronic health records, there are massive data sets available to inform our practice. Chapter 2, Nursing Value and Big Data, emphasizes the importance of data quality and analytics in leveraging Big Data to inform value-based care and the measurement of health outcomes. We need to be experts at information management and use advanced analytics to demonstrate value and create new models of care.

Rather than replacing humans, Artificial Intelligence (AI) can augment our decision-making, thus reducing cognitive burden and evolving care delivery as outlined in Chapter 3, Artificial Intelligence. Being able to use AI capabilities will allow us to take action through quick retrieval of information informed by algorithms from millions of examples. And more importantly, use of AI will return time to the caregiver so that more time is available for the human touch. AI can also aid the vulnerabilities and strengths of human performance by preventing unsafe practice. This chapter describes how predictive analytics can leverage AI to predict who will get sick, when, and how nurses should treat patients. Machine learning, another branch of AI, is also well suited for prediction using complex healthcare data, in various forms, collected from multiple sources, including large data sets.

Chapter 4, Virtual Reality, Augmented Reality, and Mixed Reality, includes a discussion of how immersive technologies such as Virtual, Augmented, and Mixed Reality will be applied in the classroom, clinical setting, and with patient education. These emerging technologies, while not yet commonplace, can be used to enhance learning practice, engage patients, and visualize a vibrant healthcare ecosystem. The author predicts that nurses will be at the forefront of keeping a delicate balance between applying these immersive technologies and the human experience.

While machine automation in healthcare has lagged compared with other industries, it is quickly catching up. Chapter 5, The Internet of Things, describes how the global economy is transitioning to a new paradigm that has been enabled through the integration of machines, platforms, and the crowd. The Internet allows us to exploit the wisdom of crowds by providing a platform to freely share information among participants. As a result, the shift to automation will likely continue at a rapid pace, improving productivity and innovating practice. Health systems must prepare for the changing roles of nurses impacted by automation.

The 21st Century Cures Act signed into law in the United States is providing impetus for the advancement and use of Precision Health and genomics in healthcare. Chapter 6, Precision Health and Genomics, describes the benefits and challenges of implementing these emerging technologies. The top three concerns identified are: (a) budget and financial, (b) integration of the data, and (c) lack of clinical expertise. Nurses and nurse informaticists have an important role to play in addressing these challenges. Research is underway focusing on nurses' ability to better understand and leverage the advances in precision health and genomics. The rapidity of discoveries and uptake of genetics are also driving the need for more competent educated nurses in academia, practice, and research.

A culture of innovation is needed for nurses to be able to leverage the tsunami of emerging technologies that are being planned and implemented in healthcare. As explored in Chapter 7, The Future of Emerging Technologies and Nursing, nurse entrepreneurs have new opportunities and a welcome voice through increasing support from nursing and health IT organizations. Nurse-led innovation is being encouraged and supported by multiple organizations, collaborations, and companies. And nurses are taking the stage as innovative leaders to advance emerging technologies that will improve healthcare for decades to come. The value of emerging technologies is their application for optimal operations that advance nursing knowledge for the best prognosis, treatments, and safe quality health outcomes.

Emerging Technologies for Nurses: Implications for Practice is an excellent resource that foreshadows the future to come. Nurses will lead this evolution, and this book is essential to help guide the way. An informative glossary is provided for each chapter along with thought-provoking questions that allow us to consider our own insights into this brave new world. I encourage you to earmark this edition as you embark on your own journey through the fascinating world of emerging technologies.

Joyce Sensmeier, MS, RN-BC, CPHIMS, FHIMSS, FAAN
Senior Advisor, Informatics
Technology and Innovation—HIMSS
Chicago, Illinois
President, Integrating the Healthcare Enterprise USA
Oak Brook, Illinois

Preface

Nursing as a profession is being transformed at lightning speed into the next decade. There is a call to nurses across the country to prepare for the National Academy of Medicine's 2020 to 2030 Future of Nursing consensus study, which will serve to recommend nursing's focus in the next decade to meet the pressing challenge to decrease health disparities in the United States. Nurses, currently numbering 4 million, are the largest population of practicing clinicians, the most significant users of health information technology (IT), and required early health IT adopters. And as the most trusted profession for 17 consecutive years, nurses are the forerunners of the process of transformation and advancement of knowledge in healthcare. For these reasons, there has never been a more exciting time to be a nurse and create the future of practice, specifically what and how to do it. We will need to do so in a more advanced fashion, by continuing to harness health IT. Utilizing new tools, processes, models, and products, including emerging technologies, will help nurses serve the Quadruple Aim—to manage populations better, decrease costs, and enhance the patient and clinician experience.

A text of this nature will be the first preview nurses will have of emerging technologies in the healthcare ecosystem. These innovations exist beyond and extend the once-revolutionary electronic health record and mobile and telehealth applications, providing a fresh glimpse of the development of these technologies and their adoption, implementation, and outcomes. An understanding of these technologies turns healthcare challenges into yet unseen opportunities for patients and nurses.

Nurses in clinical settings and nonclinical support roles face pressing clinical and operational issues in practice. With the face of health also changing rapidly, the unforeseen problem rears its head every day. To meet new and unexpected challenges requires explicit knowledge about emerging technologies—innovative, smart technologies developed to function intelligently, with more efficiency and accuracy. We all live in a society that uses innovative technologies each moment for instantaneous communication, efficiency, convenience, knowledge management, and cost savings. Yet there is currently a gap between these revolutionary technologies in nursing care delivery and administrative processes. Technological advances such as intelligent and immersive, connective, and precision technologies are now disrupting and transforming the healthcare business model. For this reason, the finer points of these technologies need understanding by practicing nurses, nursing leaders, and nurses teaching health IT and informatics courses. This textbook will serve to do that.

Within these pages, fundamentals, current and future state-specific concepts, and emerging technologies critical for the transformation of nurses' practice are examined. They are as follows:

- Healthcare and nurse innovation
- Nursing value
- Big Data
- Artificial Intelligence
- Virtual, Augmented, and Mixed Realities
- Internet of Things
- Precision Health and genomics
- The future of emerging technologies in nursing practice

How do these concepts and requirements for innovation connect? And how do emerging technologies land in nurses' hands? A clear understanding of the definition of emerging technology, along with the surfacing of healthcare as a technology industry, is required. Also important is an understanding of how technology has disrupted the healthcare industry and partnerships among vendors and health organizations to make these novel solutions available and viable in a nursing care environment. This book will give nurses a comprehensive look at how new technologies work and are applied. It will expand nurses' awareness of emerging innovations and their benefits to practice and the profession. It carefully examines the ways nurses can be a part of developing innovations and how the technologies impact value-based care and nursing value. Nurses will gain knowledge in this practical guide about how emerging technologies directly change the care they provide every day. Thus far, progress in adopting and applying these technologies in healthcare as a whole, particularly nursing, has been slow. Nursing has had little voice and visibility in developing emerging technologies and their most appropriate use. This text serves as an essential introduction for all nurses to begin using these technologies, with a collective focus on the point of care. This focus extends further than the promise of function, but with a clear strategy for operationalization.

What makes *Emerging Technologies for Nurses: Implications for Practice* unique is the examination of healthcare as a technology industry, critical divergent collaborations, and the impetus of healthcare innovation. Also, Big Data is thoughtfully utilized to provide nurse value and act as the source of all emerging technologies. The text includes details about how each emerging technology drives decision-making in tandem with the nursing process and critical thinking and how the novel technologies will move care delivery into the community and become a catalyst in health consumerism and the sharing economy. There is an unmet need for more nurse technologists who will apply their knowledge and expertise to transform critical clinical, administrative challenges in hospitals, clinically and into the community, with the intent to improve care transitions, care management, and coordination, and therefore care across the continuum. The changing roles of nurses include skilling up the workforce for advanced data analysis, advancing nursing informatics practice, and developing nurse innovators.

Both within and outside the healthcare industry, information about advanced technologies and analytics is, for the most part, gained from the media, journal articles, ebooks, White Papers, blogs, and social media pieces. They are but a substitute for a robust textbook not yet available, especially for a nursing audience. And much content about emerging technologies in healthcare is written by nonclinicians. This text will serve to meet the need for a book with a nursing focus, to add to the knowledge base about emerging technologies. The rich content will clearly explain the technologies, their applications, and the works in progress for Big Data initiatives. It serves to build on nursing informatics fundamentals to contribute to new knowledge about emerging technologies. Nurses are beginning to transform the understanding, development, adoption, and use of emerging technologies through significant work in progress globally.

Written by nurses for nurses, the text introduces all nurses in every practice setting to emerging data-driven advances in the technology industry, those that are just beginning to be used in healthcare delivery and operations today and will shape the future of nursing practice. Concise definitions and applications in case studies are provided in this text to help nurses understand the heart of modern technological innovation, emerging technologies, and, most importantly, where they fit into the healthcare landscape and how to adopt and put them into practice. The content will guide nurses in the way emerging technologies can be deployed in their healthcare settings. It bridges the gap in the availability of this content for nurse educators to teach nursing technology curriculum. This text brings together nursing experts in emerging technologies for a modern approach to information sharing with rigorous content to concisely put healthcare innovation in perspective. As an essential primer for nursing educators, the content will guide nurses in teaching about innovative health information technologies in the classroom. This text provides nurses with essential information about how data, technological advances, and innovation synergize to add value to healthcare, particularly in nursing practice, and how to use them to gain new knowledge not yet available in the nursing literature.

The main objectives of this text are to create a resource for nurses to gain in-depth knowledge about specific emerging technological healthcare innovations, increase their knowledge about how these specific technological advances improve care delivery, communicate how emerging technologies can be applied to impact care in all practice settings, direct learning about how to use these new technologies tactically, stay current and further modern nursing practice, and disseminate their use in patient care delivery and administrative processes.

A fallacy in nursing is that emerging technologies to be used in nursing practice are impending. This text provides evidence that they are already here. They need to be courageously embraced for nurses to stay current and move patient care into the next generation. *Emerging Technologies for Nurses: Implications for Practice* will be a blueprint for a new direction for nurses in health IT, and what it will become in the next decade and the 21st century. This book is intended for use as an essential source of learning, to dispel myths and highlight the vital considerations that new technology embodies for the full life cycle of the implementation of emerging technology, and to catapult nursing into a profession of industry-leading innovators and care transformers that healthcare urgently needs now and in the coming years. It is also intended to help use our invaluable skills and knowledge to develop, adopt, and apply these technologies, as well as integrate them for use now and into the next decade with the ultimate objective of meeting the needs of patients and nurses to revolutionize practice and our experience.

Whende M. Carroll

Qualified instructors may obtain access to supplementary material (Instructor's Manual and PowerPoints) by emailing textbook@springerpub.com.

Acknowledgments

I express my deep appreciation to the following experts in the health IT and advanced analytics fields:

My mentor, Joyce Sensmeier, MS, RN-BC, CPHIMS, FHIMSS, FAAN, Senior Advisor, Informatics, Technology and Innovation, HIMSS, and President, IHE, USA, for her unwavering commitment to pioneering nursing informatics, championing critical health IT initiatives, and also providing me with invaluable, constant support, guidance, and opportunities, mainly in getting this textbook started.

Muhammad Aurangzeb Ahmad, PhD, Affiliate Associate Professor, Department of Computer Science and Systems, University of Washington, Tacoma, Washington, for review of and feedback on the Artificial Intelligence chapter of this book.

Christel Anderson, Vice President, Informatics, at the Healthcare Information and Management Systems Society (HIMSS) for review of the Distributed Ledger Technology/Blockchain section at short notice.

Finally, my thanks to Joseph Morita and Hannah Hicks at Springer Publishing Company, for a shared vision for this textbook and for being responsive and easy to work with during the production of this primer on emerging technologies for all nurses and educators.

1

Emerging Technologies and Healthcare Innovation

WHENDE M. CARROLL

CHAPTER OBJECTIVES

- Define emerging technology and essential components.
- Explore the transformation of healthcare as a technology industry.
- Understand specific innovation concepts as they relate to the healthcare industry and nursing.

CONTENTS

INTRODUCTION

Existing technologies in healthcare, now commonplace, were once novel ideas, care models and devices, and new treatments. Today emerging technologies (ETs) are developed and implemented in healthcare organizations at a rapid rate. Nurses, nurse informaticists, and nurse educators should have a clear comprehension of the role of emerging technology in healthcare to optimize clinical practice. Innovation and innovators are essential to revolutionizing antiquated healthcare business models to offer new products, services, and models to modernize practice and serve the Quadruple Aim better. **Divergent collaborations** and **innovation centers** in healthcare organizations provide nurses the opportunity to be champions and early adopters and enforcers of ETs and responsible innovation, thereby improving safety and quality outcomes and promoting **health equity**. The knowledge of Nurses as innovators will further the impending need of ETs to serve the Quadruple Aim.

NURSING AND EMERGING TECHNOLOGY

Due to the pace at which **technology** is being developed, used, and is evolving, there is an expedited need to better manage patient populations (to impact quality of care and outcomes), reduce costs, improve patient satisfaction and engagement, and enhance the well-being of practicing clinicians—the four dimensions of the **Quadruple Aim** in healthcare (Bodenheimer & Sinsky, 2014; see Figure 1.1). Nurses are key players in driving these imperatives and impacting value-based care through the use of ETs.

The rapid evolution of technology shapes our world and lives. Similar to society, healthcare is now deeply connected to computers. What were once novel ideas, care models, and devices—and new treatments that influence how nurses manage care at the bedside, lead, teach, and research—are now commonplace in hospitals, clinics, virtual care environments, and in nursing education, and have improved the healthcare industry and the nursing profession. Today, technology buzzwords abound—Big Data, Artificial Intelligence (AI), Predictive Analytics and Machine Learning (ML), Virtual Reality (VR), Augmented Reality (AR), Blockchain, Precision Health, and the Internet of Things (IoT). These technologies, while not new in other industries, are increasingly being used in healthcare because of their potential

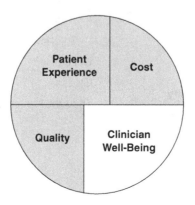

Figure 1.1 The Quadruple Aim framework.

and proven value. From a global scale to the bedside, and spaces in between, an acute need exists for a better understanding of revolutionary scientific inventions by nurses who practice, lead, and educate. Nurses hold all the aces to adopting ETs and using them in the point of care, both in the nonclinical setting and in the classroom setting. The instinct and drive to utilize and adopt technology to communicate better and complete tasks for safe, quality patient care make nurses natural innovators in practice, leadership, and education. In healthcare information technology (IT), this exceptional asset should be at the forefront to develop the necessary standards, security, equity, and policy needed to use ETs wisely.

DEFINITIONS OF EMERGING TECHNOLOGY

Understanding what makes a technology emerging is imperative to discerning past, present, and future in the development of technological innovations. Before delving into the specific ETs in healthcare, it is imperative to define what the words mean both individually and cohesively. Specifically, it is important to identify what each word represents and how they have been synthesized to become relevant in this text's focus, as well as their use to optimize nursing care delivery in the industry of healthcare. Knowledge of multiple definitions, many still evolving due to the speed at which technologies are developing and implemented, is needed to begin to explain what ETs are, as well as denote their business presence and value, complexity, misconceptions, and acceptance.

Various definitions have been put forth for ETs (Halaweh, 2013; Rotolo, Hicks, & Martin, 2015). A key challenge is that the term is, in many cases, not well defined and lacks understanding (Halaweh, 2013). When we break down the words, the term **emerging** denotes just coming into prominence. The definition of "technology" is the application of science for the use of practical purposes in a particular industry, with technology being the equipment and machinery developed from the application of that scientific knowledge. It is the tributary of knowledge addressing both engineering and applied sciences. Together these terms define the scientific inventions now used in industries across the modern landscape to help people complete tasks, communicate, make decisions, and find answers. These use cases are essential in healthcare and nursing to give patients the best possible care experience, safety, and outcomes. While definitions of the term **emerging technology** vary widely, together they form a whole expression that denotes novel scientific knowledge that is becoming less futuristic and closer to reality.

Evolving definitions of ET within the last two decades studied by Halaweh (2013) weigh the notions of Day and Schoemaker (2000), Stahl (2011), Srinivasan (2008), and the Business Dictionary ("Emerging Technologies," n.d.) and their multiple definitions posited in the last 20 years. There is a clear dissonance, with each based on the industry that uses the technology. This author asserts that the researchers have had a different view on what ETs are from the simplistic to those confined by social necessity and time frames (Halaweh, 2013).

One definition states that technology is emerging if it is not yet essential to possess by a person or user (Millea, Green, & Putland, 2005). Day and Schoemaker (2000, p. 2) and Srinivasan (2008) define ETs as "science-based innovations with the potential to create a new industry or transform an existing one." Another definition is that ETs are new technologies that are in development or will come to fruition over the next 5 to 10 years and will substantially alter major industries and society ("Emerging Technologies," n.d.). A different definition of ETs is that they must have the potential to gain social relevance within the next 10 to 15 years, with the notion that they are not only present at an early stage in development, but they have already moved beyond the purely conceptual stage (Stahl, 2011). In considering and recognizing these definitions, Halaweh (2013) asserts that ETs lack research; they do not consider social-economical and geographical contexts, including developmental costs, nor availability in certain countries as well as obvious impacts not present at the inception of technology development. These definitions of ET have come from different industries and have changed over time.

Technologies in our age are rapidly changing with new scientific-based products, services, and models at every corner. Definitions of ETs not only appear in scientific literature but also print and electronic newspaper stories, blogs, social media, and vendors. While there is variation, lack of consensus, and mass evolution of thought and theory about what makes a technology emerging, there is one standout definition that delineates aspects of what is becoming apparent scientifically in mature industries today. Rotolo et al. (2015) completed a literature review of innovative critical studies on the topic and developed a concise and meaningful term. They define "emerging technology" as "science-based machinery that is characterized by a certain degree of coherence persisting over time and with the potential to employ a considerable impact on the socio-economic domain(s) which is observed in terms of the composition of actors, institutions and patterns of relations among those, along with the concomitant knowledge production processes" (Rotolo et al., 2015). Further, these researchers assert that the most significant impact of ETs lies in the prospects of technology coming into consciousness, with the emergence phase being uncertain and ambiguous.

This definition asserts that ETs have five essential characteristics: radical novelty, fast growth, coherence, noticeable impact, and uncertainty and ambiguity (Rotolo et al., 2015), with the most prominent influence exerted by ambiguity in the nascent field of ETs. Furthering the influence of ambiguity as an apparent, divergent trait of ETs are the conflicting values and meanings attributed to them by society (Mitchell, 2007).

The defining features of ETs are complex and show that radical technological innovations at the core functioning of modern industries include, but are not limited to, furthering the improvement of practices, building sustainable products, enhancing processes, and stimulating and solidifying thoughts to advance scientific development. With this understanding of what ET means, it becomes clear that healthcare is a sector where novel technologies can be conceptualized, modernized, developed, evolved, and implemented. The use of ET improves quality and safety, decreases inefficiencies and waste, and standardizes care inclusive of all populations and communities to complement existing technologies.

Ambiguity: An Essential Factor in Emerging Technologies

Drawing on Rotolo et al.'s (2015) study and definition of ET and Adner and Levinthal's (2002) conception that the growth, development, acceptance, and adoption of new technologies is a significant factor in application, the healthcare industry is a business with multiple products, services, and models ready for disruption as ET is developed and used. It is projected that, in 2021, AI alone will generate $2.9 trillion in business revenue and recover over 6 billion hours of worker productivity in many industries (Gartner Newsroom, 2017). A movement forward with evolving and revolutionizing the business of healthcare for better physical and financial health without fluidity and divergence in thought is an obstacle for health IT users. One might argue that while there is a place for ETs in healthcare, the traits and factors that are advancing them into evidence-based practice, as previously defined—particularly ambiguity—should be avoided for safety, quality, and ethics purposes. In truth, these factors spark innovation. It is essential in an industry fraught with big problems to seek answers to solve them. In the conceptualizing, evaluating need, development, and testing phases of new technologies, diverse perspectives need to be considered, and flexibility and comfort with the unknown embraced despite incongruency. With this acceptance, the crucial questions and problems that need answers and fixing will come to light as we develop ETs in healthcare.

INNOVATION, DISRUPTION, AND HYPE

Definitions for ET present the case that novel technologies go through periods of evolution and revolution. The underlying revolutionary emergence of new technologies is often a process of shifting territories of usefulness and rapid subsequent growth in unchartered domains and how they change over time; also, the pace at which new technologies are developed, accepted, and adopted is a significant factor in technology application (Adner & Levinthal, 2002). This process requires both innovation and disruption. The terms **innovation** and **disruption** are used in multiple industries, synonymous with ETs. However, the definitions are not fully understood and can be overused to simplify the existence of new technology and a sense of blind optimism of what they can and will do, rather than their actual bearing in the marketplace.

Innovation

Today innovation refers to a novel solution that solves a problem. The technology industry and society use the term "innovation" readily. It denotes "the latest and greatest thing" that meets the needs of a rapidly evolving world dependent on technology and is used to competitively develop new ideas, inventions, and services that add value, leading many to instantly refer to these products, services, and solutions as innovation (O'Bryan, 2017). With the enormous need for radical technological solutions in banking, telecommunications, retail, and automotive industries, U.S. Commanders in Chief have put technology innovation initiatives into their policy agenda. One focus of the Obama Administration's 2016 $215 million budget for "Strategy for American Innovation" was to fund a healthcare program to advance the ET of precision health and genomics through managing and analyzing Big Data sets, furthering health IT while developing methods for increasing health data privacy (The White House, 2015). Likewise, the Trump Administration has held talks with top technology companies to begin discussions funding AI research partially aimed at the U.S. economy and the workforce (Simonite, 2018).

While innovation is what ETs stand for, the term "innovative" is what the novel idea, product, or service is, with a lack of another word for description. As a society and within industry, we speak of "innovation" readily as the endpoint and "innovative" as an adjective to describe something novel. However, in the sectors that create revolutionary solutions, innovation should be deemed instead as a series of separate proficiencies and actions (O'Bryan, 2017). Viewing innovations in this manner rather than in terms of what technology is needed will truly revolutionize and evolve novel technologies rather than generalize them by those who use the term—those who conceptualize, create, use, and fund novel solutions such as inventors, vendors, customers, and investors.

Disruption

Along with innovation, "disruption" and "disruptive" are used to describe the vast revolutionary impact innovations have on industry to effectively move the needle for solving modern customer problems and evolve business models. Disruption is an innovation that creates a new market and disrupts an existing market and traditional business practices. It explains what the innovation or ET needs to do to make it change and truly transform and modernize a marketplace. In 1995, the brainchild of innovation theory, Clayton Christensen, whose schema has been called the most influential business idea in recent years (The Economist, 2017), pronounced disruptive innovation as an arm of innovation theory, along with sustaining evolutionary and revolutionary innovations (Macfarquhar, 2012). His work asserts that disruptive innovation is one that spurs a disruption towards current existing products, market and value networks to subsequently stimulate new markets and business niches (Ab Rahman, Abdul Hamid, & Chin, 2017).

Disruption is an essential element to measure the vast change and growth innovation has in various industries. The terms together illustrate the extent to which advancements deconstruct a marketplace—and not only technology. Christensen (2018) describes disruptive innovation as "a process by which a product or service takes root initially in simple applications at the bottom of a market and then relentlessly moves up market, eventually displacing established competitors" (para. 1). Evidence of disruptive innovation over the last few decades can be seen in healthcare, where clinician communication, care delivery, standardized practices, and payer models have revolutionized the way in which healthcare is practiced. See Table 1.1 for "disruptors," those that created a novel healthcare product, service, and solution, and the "disruptee," the healthcare business models that have been transformed, and their impact on the Quadruple Aim.

As Table 1.1 represents, newer technologies in healthcare have disrupted or discontinued technologies that once were thought of as revolutionary in care delivery, such as the need for pagers to communicate among care teams, reading radiology results, and ways of documenting clinical data and information. They have evolved in the healthcare marketplace, with technological discontinuities not being a product of any particular event in the development of it, but often an evolutionary event, shifting the existing technology to a new territory where it evolves in new directions—that novel technology, or set of technologies, may be applied to a new area of application (Adner & Levinthal, 2002), in this case, healthcare.

Table 1.1 "Disruptors" and "Disruptees" and Their Effect on the Quadruple Aim in the Healthcare Industry

Disruptor	Disruptee	Business Model Transformed	Quadruple Aim Impact
Retail clinics	Primary care	Ambulatory care	Patient satisfaction
Accountable care organizations	Third-party payers	Health insurance	Controlling cost
Electronic health records	Paper charts	Clinical documentation	Clinician experience
Wearable, voice-controlled, wireless badge	Telephone or pager	Telecommunications	Clinician experience
Urgent care clinics	Emergency rooms	Hospitals	Care quality
Worksite wellness clinics	Primary care	Hospitals and clinics	Patient satisfaction
Remote monitoring	Intensive care	Hospitals	Controlling cost
Virtual care	Patient visits	Hospitals and clinics	Patient satisfaction
Robotics	Surgical care	Care delivery	Care quality
Simulation	Medical education	Education	Controlling cost
Picture archiving and communication systems	Radiology	Care delivery	Controlling cost
Advanced nurse practitioners	Physicians	Care delivery	Care quality
Mobile handheld tablets	Paper charts	Clinical documentation	Clinician experience

Disruptive Innovators

Another buzzword in modern terminology concerning new technologies and business models is the term "disruptive innovators." While disruption has a general derogatory nuance of interrupting or being problematic, the connotation has quite a different meaning for forward-thinkers in business. This term has been coined to identify key players in business and industry who elicit visionary behaviors in their approach to developing, championing, adopting, and utilizing new evolving processes and practices, by design, or intentionally using innovation theory in business to facilitate innovation. These revolutionists are the crucial resource for not only inventing ideas to diffuse and support innovation development but also to realize, further adopt, and sustain them. Five synergistic skills are distinct in disruptive innovators: having the ability to create novel products by linking ideas previously unconnected to solve problems; persistent questioning and observing and being fervently experimental (Dyer, Gregersen, & Christensen, 2011). Disruptors harness these skills to think differently and bring new products, services, and models to fruition. In light of the innovations in healthcare, disruptive innovators certainly exist in the industry. As ET evolves rapidly, visionaries, inventors, implementors, and researchers with these traits will change evidence-based practice and be relentless to revolutionize the future of the health of individuals and all populations not only at the macro-level but through further innovations at the point of care (Case Study 1.1).

CASE STUDY 1.1

A PRIMARY CARE GAME CHANGER: VERA WHOLE HEALTH

Disruptive healthcare delivery models surfacing around the country are serving a need for healthcare that focuses on time savings and convenience to maximize cost savings and patient-centered health engagement for improved outcomes. The exposure to a new model that provides a supplemental option for flexible full healthcare services for both employers and employees is beginning to change traditional primary and specialty care and payer models—direct-to-employer advanced primary care (Patient-Centered Primary Care Collaborative, 2018).

Vera Whole Health, a Seattle-based company offering on-site and near-worksite advanced primary care centers, is changing models of healthcare delivery as an alternative primary and specialty care provider. With the high cost of urgent care center, emergency department, and specialty care visits in today's value-based care landscape, this new model of care delivery provides holistic care to employees in a medical home structure to increase employee health engagement and lowers employee out-of-pocket healthcare costs, as well as costs to employers. The innovative care model for full-service on-site advanced primary care works by charging an employer a per member per month (PMPM) fee for care services in addition to employee health benefits, without co-pays, deductibles, or additional fees to access Vera's advanced primary care centers. The employee or plan-funded model removes third-party payers from these care transactions and transforms the traditional health insurance framework for primary care and specialty care, saving employers a significant amount of money with centrally located care centers offering multiple health services (R. Schmid, personal interview, December 19, 2018).

In today's "now economy" healthcare expectations, Vera Whole Health's model meets healthcare consumers' needs, improving their overall care experience. With Vera's board-certified providers, wellness coaches, telehealth services, and website portal and app, patients can be seen sooner for all types of conditions in one care center to circumvent the need for expensive urgent and specialty care. The flat fee

(continued)

CASE STUDY 1.1 (*continued*)

to employers for full-service primary care encounters includes preventative health screenings and biometric testing for employee wellness incentives. And, in conjunction with the provision of acute care services for minor injuries and illnesses, travel medicine, immunizations and pharmacy, occupational health, vision, rehabilitation, behavioral health services, and basic disease management (Vera Whole Health, 2019), this model is a game changer in a fragmented healthcare system.

Leading the direct-to-employer primary care provider marketplace in the Western United States, Vera Whole Health employs physicians and nurse practitioners in a patient-centered medical home care delivery framework. They offer wellness coaching for health behavior modification, ensuring whole person-centered care and enhanced patient health engagement. The medical home model enables the company to implement a population health management strategy, to track and build care plans for all employees, and target the sickest patients to address their essential needs to improve health outcomes. Vera's comprehensive care center model supports better access to care with same-day appointments and timely follow-up encounters which are becoming difficult for many patients to adequately secure with primary and specialty providers, mitigating costly emergency and specialty care services for considerable savings to employers.

In Western Washington, the City of Kirkland launched its Vera Whole Healthcare centers to optimize its employee health benefits strategy in 2015 to decrease healthcare costs and improve long-term health outcomes for their employees. Vera's adjunct care delivery service enabled the employer to achieve a 90% employee engagement rate in 12 months, leading to a 25% reduction in claims and 15% net savings in overall healthcare costs, and decreasing the city's number of employee claims trend within 2 years (Vera Whole Health, 2018). Furthering their disruptive model throughout the United States, Vera Whole Health now has 19 care centers in eight states, and they are partnering with Blue Cross and Blue Shield of Kansas City (Blue KC) to operate advanced primary care centers under the name Spira Care Centers in Missouri. Spira Care is a combined primary care and health insurance offering available exclusively to eligible Blue KC members for the care centers in the state. The partnership is a sign of persistent healthcare model transformation between payers and worksite advanced primary care centers to further the creating of new, collaborative care models that prioritize primary and specialty care for employee health engagement to improve lasting health outcomes and to lower staggering healthcare costs around the country (R. Schmid, personal interview, December 19, 2018).

Innovation and Hype

As nurses learn about the terms associated with ETs, how they revolutionize business models, the importance of customers' demands, and expectation of ETs is clear. The notion of ETs is stimulating both to the ear and imagination, but the terms themselves can be overused. The terms "innovation," "innovative," "disruption," and "disruptive" may lead us to believe that anything is possible with ETs and that anyone in the realm is an expert. This notion can result in the hype and lofty expectations about what ETs are and what they can do for us (Lucker, Hogan, & Sniderman, 2018). **Hype** can be defined as extravagant or intensive publicity or promotion. The attention in the news and social media related to innovations, including vendor advertisements, blogs, and articles that stop at addressing the function of ETs, can create a false reality of their use and outcomes. In truth, the creation of disruptive innovations takes time, as they are dependent on the development of ideas, needed use cases, the abilities and numbers of skilled developers, and the success of their utility. These innovations are developed rapidly, possibly too quickly, based on customer demands and modern societies' "now economy." Inflated promises and ideals of the purpose and expectation of how ETs will serve us can lead to failure as well, and those can many times go unnoticed. Many developers of novel technologies claim to have the latest and greatest product, and many people erroneously refer to themselves as "disruptive innovators." They merely speak of the promise of innovation and what it may do for nurses without proving its value and using innovation theory to disseminate it. However, talk and speculation are not enough. Diffusion of hype through skepticism and education is imperative. Valuable outcomes of ETs can become certain, given time, market demand, and proof of actual return on investment. Having the right mind to cultivate innovations and disseminate them will move us from hype to reality in the creation and use of ETs.

HEALTHCARE AS A TECHNOLOGY INDUSTRY

Today all companies are technology companies, as no business can develop, market, or deliver services and products and introduce new models without it (Stone, 2017). Healthcare as a business is no exception, one where ET abounds with some of the top 10 technology companies (Stoller, 2018), including Apple, Samsung, and Microsoft, aiming to lead disruptive innovation in the industry (Huynh, 2018). Apple, Inc., known for desktop and handheld computers, music services, and smartphones, is working on enhancing the usability of its ever-evolving consumer-facing products to mimic medical devices. Several of their new products and devices are aimed at tracking diseases, sharing and trending clinical health data, detecting abnormal patient vital signs and physical movements, and allowing payment directly from their devices for medical services (CB Insights, 2017). Samsung, with a historically enormous presence in telecommunications, home electronics, and household appliances sectors, has a health division also focused on consumer wearables to enhance the patient experience. Their immersive device offering uses VR to distract patients from pain during medical procedures, diagnose and manage mental health and neurological disorders, and provide therapeutic rehabilitation technology to improve care quality and cost (Muoio, 2018). Microsoft, the world's largest microchip maker, also aims to be a leader in healthcare innovation. By leveraging of HIPAA-compliant cloud computing for data management and security, the company now offers predictive analytics and ML aimed at improved precision health, enhanced clinical decision support, and reduction of clinical documentation for healthcare providers (Bresnick, 2018b). Together, these three top technology companies are moving into the healthcare marketplace to offer digital health solutions aimed at a full-service connected care continuum for the patient focused on health and well-being while reducing costs, managing populations, and improving healthcare to improve the clinician experience. The collaboration between researchers and health systems can have a high impact on value-based care and the Quadruple Aim.

While large-scale IT companies are getting the most attention in their disruptive products, services, and prototypes in the healthcare space as they attempt to transform it with their business models, smaller healthcare companies are cited as true disruptors in the healthcare IT sector. CVS Health's pharmacy services; genetics-based testing companies including 23andMe, Color, Veritas Genetics, and Helix; and high-risk patient care management apps Glooko and Emocha Mobile Health are among these healthcare technology companies (Fast Company, 2018). These retail businesses and smaller companies are truly patient-centered, with a focus on patient engagement and connected health to serve all arms of the Quadruple Aim, working to deliver healthcare services, products, and models that modernize care delivery based on healthcare provider and consumer demand, thereby enabling better data transfer, customer convenience, and precision care.

In 2015, CVS opened an innovation lab to develop services for its customers to enable smartphone text reminders for refills and barcoding prescription technology at the point of service for faster, more convenient processing of new and refilled prescriptions (Castellanos, 2017). The demand for company offerings of 23andme, Color, Veritas Genetics, and Helix stems from a mass market of consumers curious about inherited health and what they can do with the knowledge of it. These companies offer direct-to-consumer testing kits that analyze DNA for ancestry discovery, disease hereditary testing, and disease prediction, without a healthcare provider's order (National Institutes of Health—U.S. National Library of Medicine, 2018). Affordable, comparative to laboratory testing, self-testing kits offer genetic data for personal use to further genomic research for rare and common conditions such as cancer and heart disease with the intent to enable consumers to understand their health risks better and use the data for personal, preemptive, and precision health (Bresnick, 2018a). Glooko, a diabetes care management app-driven tool that interfaces with many home glucose monitors, insulin pumps, and exercise trackers, sends patient data directly to his or her healthcare providers, with a web interface that shows the trends of the patient's glucose levels and makes recommendations for diet food and exercise to help manage the chronic condition (Lovett, 2018). Emocha is a mobile app that aims to monitor medication adherence in high-risk populations including those with HIV, tuberculosis, and hepatitis C through video directly observed therapy (VDOT; Wicklund, 2018). A study of TB patients using the Emocha app resulted in increased medication compliance, with researchers recommending the platform for utilization in medication management of high-risk patients requiring regularly scheduled therapy to improve patient-centered care and cost savings (Holzman, Zenilman, & Shah, 2018).

Partnering for Healthcare Innovation

Because hospitals, clinics, and their administration lack the innovation leadership, know-how, inspiration, and ideas to disrupt their healthcare system business models effectively to improve value-based care, many are looking for healthcare technology industry innovators to partner with them. This emerging trend partners organizations with big technology players and **start-ups**—new small companies focused on a specific industry business problem to solve: to spearhead innovation (Gaskell, 2017). Together, healthcare organizations and leading-edge technology innovators aim to disrupt their business models by collaborating to rapidly develop products and services to transform patient care with the intent of improving quality and safety, and reducing costs. In tandem, resources pooled from these divergent collaborations foster new ways of thinking to conceptualize, build, test, and implement novel technology, and sustain innovation within the healthcare organization (Zand, 2017). This radical approach is successful when talent outside of a healthcare organization brings ideas and an innovative spirit for the invention of using technology to its fullest extent and reaching even further beyond to invent new models and use existing technology in different ways (Gaskell, 2017). In many cases, this has led to the establishment of innovation centers within healthcare organizations focusing on multiple innovation projects that use ETs as a cornerstone of new products, services, and models. They have also resulted in establishing health-focused start-ups and **spin-offs** in healthcare IT—organization, university, or research institutions who develop their own companies and businesses. See Figure 1.2 for a depiction of how these relationships work.

Healthcare Innovation Centers Advancing Emerging Technologies

With disruptive innovation now common in the healthcare industry, the fruits of divergent collaborations between vendors—the big IT players, and start-ups and spin-offs—and healthcare organizations are essential to catalogue and disseminate

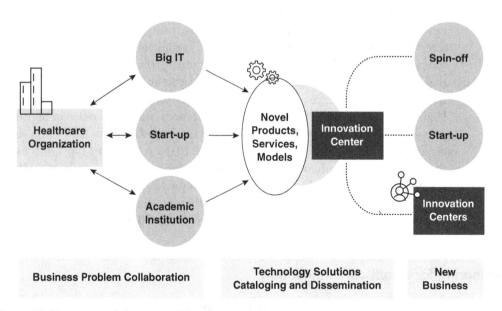

Figure 1.2 The process of divergent collaborations.
IT, information technology.

innovation knowledge, products, and processes to hospitals and healthcare systems who need education to build innovations and disrupt business models.

In a survey conducted by the American Hospital Association (AHA), close to three-quarters of large healthcare organizations have either built an innovation center or have plans to build one soon (Sullivan, 2017). These centers are becoming businesses themselves, patenting their inventions developed in the labs for mass distribution. Multiple entities, from healthcare organizations to medical health IT associations, have embarked on the journey to establish hotspots for the creation and dissemination of innovative solutions and knowledge across the globe.

The Cleveland Clinic, one of the pioneers in the creation of healthcare innovation laboratories, has had significant success with its innovation center, Cleveland Clinic Innovations (CCI), established in 2000. Since then, with divergent collaborations and a strong commitment and culture dedicated to innovation within their institution, they have invented over a thousand licenses and issued patents and created over 40 spin-offs (Cleveland Clinic Innovations, n.d.). The CCI now holds innovation events, summits, and presents awards nationally for healthcare innovations—medical devices, new treatments and procedures, and uses of ETs, such as AI and VR, and precision health.

The AHA has followed the healthcare industry's transformation trajectory and established the Center for Health Innovation in 2018 (AHA, n.d.). The AHA intends to use innovation to test new payment and delivery models, better utilize IT and data, and develop the leadership skills and competencies necessary to transform healthcare by identifying novel ideas and opportunities and implementing them (Slabodkin, 2018). The intent is to assist hospital and health systems to build new advances at scale to transform value-based care.

The Healthcare Information and Management Systems Society (HIMSS), a global, cause-based, nonprofit advisory organization that supports the transformation of health through the application of information and technology (HIMSS, n.d.-a), has also developed a proprietary innovation lab. Built to host events focused on developing health information technologies, the Center is a hub to bring IT industry leaders together to convene and confer about healthcare innovation at all levels of maturity to educate the public about disruptive technologies (HIMSS, n.d.-b). In 2018, they acquired Healthbox, a leader in health innovation consulting to further the abilities of healthcare organizations by developing the tools to bring healthcare innovations into their systems and help manage funding for disruptive technology projects (Sullivan, 2018).

Conscientious Innovation

In healthcare, clinicians are held accountable for promoting safety and quality (The National Academies of Sciences, Engineering, and Medicine, 2018) and mitigating implicit bias in the care of patients (The Joint Commission, 2016). Health IT that revolutionizes the way we practice and impact people, populations, and communities needs the same layer of safety, quality, objectivity, and fairness in the advancement of disruptive innovations such as ETs. With the new reality and focus on divergent collaborations that expedite new technology-based products, services, and models, careful consideration should be given to why, how, when, and where we develop new scientific advancements (Browne, 2018). The real value of technical development, transparency, and interpretability of functionality, truthful marketing, and proof of return on investment of ETs is imperative to the ultimate end users—patients, clinicians, administrators, and society at large. Developing innovations to disrupt business models with the aim of "Rush to Market" services, products, and new models that serve the Quadruple Aim can be misleading, and not representative of those intended. In the conception, feasibility, assessment, development, testing, and validity phases of disruptive innovations, the human elements of design, usability, and experience need close consideration (Lehoux et al., 2014).

If ambiguity is an essential component of novel technologies, as is the speed at which they are developed and implemented, essential societal fragments get forgotten and lost in an inventor's and developer's consciousness and approach, leading to an explosion of ethical concerns. Human representation, well-being, impact, and accessibility need careful reflection during the conception, evaluation, development, testing, employment, marketing, and research of ETs.

U.S. Food and Drug Administration: Taking Steps to Protect Patient Risk With Medical Device Innovation

In 2016, the U.S. Food and Drug Administration (FDA) founded the patient and clinic-focused National Evaluation System for Health Technology (NEST) initiative, aimed at the medical device industry, whose mission is to leverage the experiences of patients to inform decisions about medical device safety, effectiveness, and quality to promote public health and support optimal patient care (Daniel, Colvin, Silcox, McClellan, & Bryan, 2016). In 2018, the FDA announced the first device safety pilot using NEST would focus on women's health, specifically to develop a surveillance system using data to monitor the effects of the implantable devices to enhance post-market safety (FDA, 2018a). That same year, the FDA's Center for Devices and Radiological Health (CDRH) released the Medical Device Safety Action Plan: Protecting Patients, Promoting Public Health (FDA, 2018b), which outlines how the agency will incite innovation to enhance safety, detect safety risks earlier, and keep clinicians and patients better informed. The plan modernizes methods to improve measures for the safe use of medical devices while continuing to create more efficient pathways to bring lifesaving devices to patients, with the vision to create a medical device safety net that supports innovation of new products that are safer, more effective, and address unmet medical needs (FDA, 2018b).

Health Disparities and Emerging Technology

Community and cultural impact differ in the onslaught of disruptive innovation and can be a victim of untoward outcomes, neglectful of receiving the benefits of disruptive innovation. The influence on society requires deep reflection. As we move forward with our rapid developments, transparency, unrelenting testing, substantial inquiry, and scrutiny are needed. The fruits of these healthcare innovations must be inclusionary and reach all of society for optimal outcomes. Cultural and ethnic diversity that is forgotten makes ETs moot and unforeseen consequences will abound. For instance, the data that feed ET must be inclusionary of all demographics and free of bias—aimed to represent and serve all populations and demographics equally (Gershgorn, 2018), as it determines the way that people are, or are not, affected by innovation (Adner & Levinthal, 2002). In healthcare, intangible elements such as socioeconomics and the way that people present, perform, and live in their environment cannot be discounted in the development and use of technology; currently, people are increasingly trying to collect and analyze these elements (Correa-de-Araujo, 2017). Through successfully including these structures that can now solely be physically assessed and managed through human interaction, accurate representation and benefits of innovation have a better chance of being realized for all.

THE SOCIAL DETERMINANTS OF HEALTH

In data, the features at the core of ET functionality, unknown public health factors and the **Social Determinants of Health** (SDoH), are elements needing careful inclusion in the inception and implementation of novel innovations. One focus of the use of ET should be health equity versus health disparity. Given the differences in health status globally, populations should be represented and targeted in the life cycle of ET implementation. This divide exists, as evident in the different ways in which people live in their environment—which is difficult to collect in clinical systems (Correa-de-Araujo, 2017) and present clinically—access healthcare, and receive treatment. In the development of ET, another gap exists, in the people represented in data sets at the center of ET development and receiving its benefits. Data that represent and affect people's lives derived from the non-medical drivers of a patient's health can improve quality of care and enrich the utility of so-called intelligent machines (Ready, 2017), such as those used for machine-driven ETs in healthcare. Much of what happens in people's health, which lies outside of clinician and administrative data collection from electronic health records (EHRs) and administrative claims data, is critical to collect, analyze, and be represented in the data that feed ET. Because of this, the likelihood of health disparities increases in the use, access of, and deriving benefit of emerging technologies. This is the reason the precise representative of all populations in health IT systems is imperative.

The SDoH are mostly responsible for health inequities—the unfair and avoidable differences in health status seen within and between countries. They are the conditions in which people are born, grow, live, work, and age—the circumstances determined by the distribution of money, power, and resources at global, national, and local levels (World Health Organization, 2018). Additional conditions, such as where people learn, play, and worship, affect a wide range of health, functioning, and quality-of-life outcomes and risks. The patterns of social engagement and a sense of security and well-being affected by where people live (Centers for Disease Control and Prevention, 2018) give us a better understanding of health status. Because of the difficulty in collecting these social and environmental factors in the form of data, a greater divide exists to portray the finite characteristics of all populations in healthcare accurately.

DATA AND HEALTH EQUITY

The use of Big Data and data science methods to advance the field of symptoms management is in its infancy (Correa-de-Araujo, 2017). Related to the development of technology is the greater recognition of what's involved in getting and keeping people healthy, rather than what happens in the clinical system (Ready, 2017). The exclusion of age, gender, race, sexual orientation, and culture in accurately determining a patient's health status presents a risk of misrepresenting access and inclusion in data sets and therefore skews the outcomes, inclusion, and accessibility to healthcare services and treatments at the population level and point of care.

For clinicians, health disparities and exclusion of specific populations from accessing ETs cannot be paused for future ethicists to address. Health IT researchers, such as those studying AI, are now presenting their healthcare technologies as viable for providing both second opinions and alternative options in care delivery (Gershgorn, 2018). This fact makes it imperative to ensure policies and regulations are in place to include all populations equally in the development and testing phases of ETs, contrary to the reality today.

NURSES: CATALYSTS IN EMERGING TECHNOLOGY DEVELOPMENT

Serving the Quadruple Aim is the goal of using ETs. To bear fruit, nurses must be a part of creating novel scientific machinery, by inventing new products and services, and also influencing the design and use of new care models. Historically, nurse practice was based on standardization of care based on policies, procedures, and protocols, which led to limited opportunities for innovation. Today, a chance to transform practice lies in using ETs to better care for patients, decrease healthcare costs, and enhance patient experience and engagement while improving clinician well-being to disrupt the healthcare industry.

A Call to Action for Nurse Innovation

There has been a summons for nurses to be partners within their health organizations to advance healthcare innovation. In the 2010 Institute of Medicine's (IOM's) landmark report *The Future of Nursing, Leading Change, Advancing Health*, national healthcare leaders and policy makers put forth specific guidance for nurses to further the profession through the recommendation of evolving education standards, workforce designs, practice models, and the use of health IT. The specific proposal for promoting the conception, development, adoption, and effective utilization of innovative technologies is to "expand opportunities for nurses to lead and diffuse collaborative improvement efforts" (IOM, 2010, p. 11). Further, the report asserts that this should occur through healthcare organizations engaging nurses to collaborate with health IT developers and manufacturers in the design, development, purchase, implementation, and evaluation of medical devices and products (IOM, 2010, p. 11), and that "These entities should also provide opportunities for nurses to diffuse successful practices" (p. 11). Regarding innovation and new care models, the report stresses a necessary industry-wide action is "changing the way we think"—discarding our current models of work and replacing them with something altogether different—and health organization leaders need to foster cultures of innovation and build effective teams to do their jobs, requiring drastic culture change and transformational leadership (p. 417; Case Study 1.2).

CASE STUDY 1.2

A LEADER'S ROADMAP TO NURSE-LED INNOVATION

A conversation is beginning about nursing innovations as it connects to the future of clinical practice. We are in the infancy of nurse innovation and are beginning to understand what it is, how to harness it, and how nurse leaders must respond to involve nursing in understanding and to operationalize innovation concepts to nurses in clinical settings for the dissemination of evidence-based practice (Davidson, Weberg, Porter-O'Grady, & Malloch, 2017). The advancement of prioritizing innovation strategy for implementation of disruption in healthcare organizations is trickle-down. Nursing leaders across the care continuum require comprehension of innovation concepts to further great ideas from nurses that enhance patient care delivery, whether it is encouraging nurses to the development of new devices, methods to improve clinical and administrative workflows, or evidence-based practice frameworks. Nurses on the frontlines of patient care must be free to create novel products, processes, and models, and a robust leadership paradigm that is well versed and committed to an innovative spirit will do so (Davidson et al., 2017).

To advance innovative change, nurse leaders must understand what differentiates innovative healthcare organizations from others and puts them ahead of the curve in transforming care, in forward-thinking nursing environments—clinical and nonclinical professional—advancing innovation. Nursing leaders' guidance and enablement for all nurses to be disruptive encourages and furthers nurses' innovation knowledge, beyond the bedside and into shared-governance committees and risk management and quality improvement teams that will own and guide transformation in care through team interaction that stimulates the innovation process. Nurse leaders can create settings to learn about and adopt innovation concepts and institute them appropriately where care is planned, taught, and delivered by nurses who develop policies and procedures, as well as project, manage, and engage in operational excellence. These departments are many times nurse-led—they are the teams in a healthcare organization that identify issues in care, understand change management, and can sustain new practices that result from innovation projects (Carroll, n.d.).

An actionable, beneficial nurse innovation leadership guide published in 2016, *The Innovation Road Map: A Guide for Nurse Leaders* by Cianelli, Clipper, Freeman, Goldstein, and Wyatt, lends nurse leaders a deep dive into the components, characteristics, and collaboration needed in high-functioning innovative healthcare organizations focused on nurse-led innovation, and how leaders encourage the use of innovative concepts in evidence-based practice.

Leading Nurses in Innovative Healthcare Organizations		
Characteristics	Divergent thinking	Leaders encourage different vs. linear thinking, and the behaviors consisting of trying something completely new and different from current practices, in a safe environment for nurseswhere leaders view failure as opportunities for learning.
	Risk-taking	
	Failure tolerance	

(continued)

CASE STUDY 1.2 (*continued*)

Leading Nurses in Innovative Healthcare Organizations		
Characteristics (*continued*)	Agility and flexibility	Leaders enable nurses' ability to adapt quickly to rapidly developing trends and changing market conditions, and act based on their knowledge and judgment, within their full scope of practice as defined by existing professional, regulatory, and organizational rules.
	Autonomy and freedom	
Components	Employee feedback	Leaders promote the impetus for change by allowing nurses' input, both positive and negative, to develop ideas for transformation, and hire courageous nurses and executive leaders with keen imagination and vision, who mentor and provide recognition to stimulate creativity and challenge the status quo. Leaders identify and safeguard engagement activities and committees that spark and feed nurses' creative spirits and identify early adopters and champions for transformation, to enlist help to encourage widespread innovative approaches such as teaching design thinking and concepts of invention to solve standard nursing problems. Leaders provide nurses with exclusive technology resources that allow for idea-to-concept discovery through access to scholarly literature databases and hands-on learning-labs and advocate for the use of transformation methodologies focused on observation, ideation, rapid prototyping, user feedback, iteration, and implementation, keeping the end user in mind while creating and applying innovations.
	Role filling	
	Role modeling	
	Employee engagement	
	Education	
	Protected time	
	Technological support	
	Rewards	
	IDEO methodology	
	Budgeting	
	Leadership	

(*continued*)

CASE STUDY 1.2 (*continued*)

Leading Nurses in Innovative Healthcare Organizations		
Components (*continued*)		Leaders, at all levels in the organization, are visible, vocal, and active role models for nurse inventiveness, and control innovation expenses that, while not producing a financial return on investment, have a lasting cultural impact for positive change in the work environment.
Collaboration	Unlikely and diverse team members	Leaders support nursing team collaboration by including enthusiastic and risk-tolerant, uncertain, and varying members committed to a common goal to encourage productive interaction, taking into account all perspectives and backgrounds to see a project to completion. Leaders promote a fun atmosphere to stimulate creativity and allow rest during innovative work sessions, developing nurses' aptitude for novel thinking to make the collaborative process more inventive and efficient.
	Productive interaction	
	Play pauses and breaks	
	Skill set development	

The Power to Transform Care

Nurses are highly skilled and well-trained innovators, who can lead the revolution to transform care through the use of ETs. With a keen ability to create new ways to deliver safer, quality care, improve health outcomes, and enhance patient experience through the acquisition of technology and strategizing its use, nurses are well positioned to be the pioneers of new ways to ignite change and continue to be the foundation of organizational stability and growth (McGonigle & Mastrian, 2017, p. 111). For care delivery to indeed evolve, nurses as knowledge workers must disrupt practice patterns that diminish useful results and embrace a collective goal to improve care through process redesign and use of IT and advanced analytics (HIMSS, 2011). **Clinical practice transformation** moves "beyond the form and function of nursing practice as we know it today by boldly advancing the redesign of clinical processes and being open to emerging transformative possibilities within society and healthcare through the use of technology" (Nagle & Yetman, 2009, p. 2).

Clinical transformation involves assessing and continually improving patient care delivery at all levels in healthcare. It occurs when existing inefficient or less effective care models are rejected, and a group or organization embraces a common goal of patient safety, clinical outcomes, and quality care through process redesign and technology. By expertly blending people, processes, and technology, clinical transformation occurs across facilities, departments, and clinical fields of expertise (HIMSS, 2011). With this in mind, clinical practice transformation, led by nurse knowledge workers, is possible with the adoption and use of ETs, such as AI, VR, and the IoT. Nurses have an immense opportunity to guide their application in evidence-based practice for multiple use cases. Combining ET with significant clinical knowledge, and through understanding and implementing innovation skills, nurses have the pull to bring this to fruition and add value to clinical practice by leveraging it (Case Study 1.3).

CASE STUDY 1.3

PUTTING IT ALL TOGETHER HELPSY HEALTH: A VISIONARY NURSE-LED START-UP FOR CANCER SYMPTOM MANAGEMENT AND REFERRAL

Across all industries, new companies are exploding on the scene at a rapid pace to develop new services, products, and processes designed to disrupt current business models and leverage technology to challenge the status quo. Healthcare start-ups are no exception. Clinician-led companies are identifying patient-centered direct care and administrative payment problems and are quickly developing innovative health IT solutions to fix them. With a focus on care quality, patient experience, engagement and satisfaction, and reducing healthcare costs, hundreds of companies have set out to meet the dimensions of the Quadruple Aim—the modern framework designed to improve healthcare delivery.

Helpsy Health, a Silicon Valley-based, nurse-led healthcare start-up, had developed an artificial intelligence-based solution explicitly focused on improving patient care quality and safety and reducing medical costs. The company's comprehensive symptom management software platform for cancer patients was established in 2016 to meet the need for vital support for patients experiencing physical and emotional cancer symptoms that busy providers cannot. The company's vision of the future is one where cancer patients, experts, and treatment centers are able to benefit from and provide high-touch care quality and increase care team efficiencies. Their aim is to leverage technology to enable patients to better engage and make their care choices and have better, more timely access to cancer experts and resources. Their patient-centered software platform is designed to significantly reduce these barriers to care and financial concerns through ongoing support from nurses and interprofessional care teams, thoughtful use of technology for easier connectivity to provide continuity of care, education, and reminders, where healthcare organizations are limited financially.

(continued)

CASE STUDY 1.3 (*continued*)

In its inception, Helpsy Health identified evidence-based critical quality, safety, and financial issues related to cancer care. The company found that 90% of patients with complex conditions such as cancer experience preventable adverse events due to lack of patient education, continuity of care, and treatment adherence, with each event costing approximately $20,000 per patient per event; 77% of this cost is passed onto insurance companies and self-insured employers, resulting in high costs to all (S. Agarawal, personal communication, June 9, 2019). As hospitals and cancer centers aim to provide critical, continuous follow-up care, cancer patients need to manage side effects and continuing symptoms; with the 2015 Commission on Cancer mandating cancer centers provide survivorship care, cancer providers continue to lose over $50,000 per year to maintain comprehensive care programs (S. Agarawal, personal communication, June 9, 2019). Because insurance companies cover 1 hour for care planning per patient visit, cancer care management can be arduous and expensive, and barriers remain to successful survivorship programs that are detrimental to cancer survivors' lives.

Armed with this knowledge, Helpsy Health has set out on a mission to create a futuristic care delivery and payment model to help patients, care delivery teams, and cancer centers use technology to bridge care gaps and improve efficiencies by offering critical symptom-focused, personalized patient care plans. Their innovative, customizable, and HIPAA-compliant platform supports cancer patients in searching for options based upon their condition and individual needs and in collaboration with healthcare teams, and ensures effective results (Agarawal, 2018). Their novel solution offers a comprehensive, whole-health symptom management and navigation platform that addresses cancer patients' physical, emotional, and social needs to create a whole-healthcare plan for patient symptoms, utilizing 20,000 recommendations and 5,000 resources across 20 social determinant categories, in real time (Helpsy Health, 2019a).

The Helpsy Health software platform offers a patient a portal in addition to a smart device app that connects to virtual services to access and develop symptom management and Quality-of-Life Care Plans (Helpsy Health, 2019b). The care plan includes treatment education, symptom management, medication adherence monitoring, and reminders, and provides community resources to improve care coordination during and after cancer treatments. At the core of the cancer care plans is the combination of evidence-based therapies from multiple modalities including nursing, social work, nutrition, and mindfulness following guidelines proposed by the NCCN, ONS, the ASCO, and other professional organizations. Ongoing symptom and adverse event management platforms remind patients of upcoming visits and testing, direct patients to in-network services, and provide continuous active and passive monitoring through wearables and EHRs. For interprofessional care teams, the online cloud-based, EHR-integrated solution enables efficient checking and adjustments of the patients' care plans throughout successive treatment phases to promote patient care team connectedness and improve patient engagement. The platform also risk-stratifies cancer patients using clinical decision support to alert care teams of high-risk patients and patient decline, supporting actionable, efficient, precision care, and decision-making. Platform analytics provide insights for quality, performance, and cost metrics, and

(*continued*)

CASE STUDY 1.3 (*continued*)

collect patient satisfaction scores and once manual cancer screening tools such as the PRO, Distress, and RWE virtually (Helpsy Health, 2019b).

Early studies of their platform in collaboration with the National Institutes of Health and the University of California San Francisco (UCSF) provided evidence of the need for a cancer symptom management solution. An unmet need supported cancer care teams to complete higher value tasks and improve patient experience and empower cancer patients and their care partners to have continuous clarity, guidance, support, and assistance between provider visits. As demonstrated in clinical studies of the Helpsy Health solution (S. Agarawal, personal communication, June 9, 2019), patients using the intelligent symptom management platform and referral service improved by 30% to 70% and quality of life improved by 14% to 78%. When investigating cost savings models, Helpsy Health's solution saved insurance companies $5,000 per patient during active treatment. For value-based care organizations, conserving resources and minimizing costs enabled health providers to implement high-quality care through provider referrals to the patient-centered service (S. Agarawal, personal communication, June 9, 2019).

Helpsy Health's desire to facilitate the emergence of a new healthcare ecosystem by connecting experts, patients, and centers using its intelligent, online, customizable, comprehensive survivorship care program that cancer patients have been struggling to find, and cancer centers have been struggling to provide, continues to grow in the marketplace. Nurse-led innovations and start-ups such as Helpsy Health empower nurses to develop and use novel technologies to transform care through software platforms to guide patients, care partners, and care teams virtually, with health IT devices, products, and services critical to modern healthcare delivery in ambulatory and virtual settings. Health IT start-ups, such as Helpsy Health, are changing how nurses provide care using emerging technologies to improve complex patient care and move the healthcare industry further to meet the Quadruple Aim.

CONCLUSION

ET—scientific-based machinery with the characteristics of radical novelty, fast growth, coherence, noticeable impact, uncertainty and ambiguity introduced into practice—is developing and being implemented at lightning speed. As healthcare evolves into technology business, strong collaborations are occurring to revolutionize the products, services, and models to serve the Quadruple Aim successfully. Innovation, the critical component to further technology development, must be brought to the forefront by forward-thinking leaders and in a way that significantly alters the industry. ETs should be disseminated through centers that excel and are successful at cultivating innovation. The life cycle of ETs must take a conscientious approach with safety and inclusion of all populations in the conception, development, testing, validating, and marketing to prove efficacy and return on investment. Nurses, nurse informaticists, and nurse educators using innovation concepts with significant clinical knowledge are uniquely positioned as catalysts in the development, adoption, and utilization of ETs in transformative ways, to serve the Quadruple Aim. At the forefront of moving ETs into all settings, including hospitals, clinics, virtual environments, and the classroom, nurses will be the purveyors of ETs as they permeate healthcare today and in the future.

GLOSSARY

Clinical Practice Transformation: Going beyond the form and function of current nursing practice by advancing the redesign of clinical processes and being open to evolving possibilities within society and healthcare.

Emerging: Just coming into prominence.

Emerging Technology: Science-based machinery characterized by a certain degree of coherence persisting over time and with the potential to considerably impact society, interacting actors, and institutions and patterns of relations. The concomitant knowledge production processes have five characteristics: radical novelty, fast growth, coherence, noticeable impact, and uncertainty and ambiguity.

Disruption: New ways of doing things that disrupt or overturn traditional business methods and practices.

Divergent Collaboration: Healthcare organizations and leading-edge technology innovators collaborating to rapidly develop products and services to disrupt existing business models and transform patient care with the intent of improving quality and safety, as well as reducing costs.

Health Equity: Unfair and avoidable differences in health status seen within and between countries.

Hype: Extravagant or intensive publicity or promotion.

Innovation: New ideas, inventions, and services developed for products, models, and solutions.

Innovation Center: Entities within healthcare and technology organizations focusing on projects that use innovation as a cornerstone of developing new products, services, and models.

Quadruple Aim: A framework developed to improve health through managing patient populations, reducing costs, improving patient satisfaction and engagement, and enhancing the well-being of practicing clinicians.

Social Determinants of Health (SDoH): Conditions where people live, learn, work, and play concerning a wide range of health risks and outcomes.

Spin-off: Companies who base businesses on products or technology initially developed in an umbrella organization, university, or research institution.

Start-up: Small companies focused on solving a specific industry business problem and spearheading innovation.

Technology: Application of science for the use of practical purposes in a particular industry, with technology being the equipment and machinery developed from the application of that scientific knowledge.

THOUGHT-PROVOKING QUESTIONS

1. Which aspects of the emerging technologies definition are most relevant in your work setting? How might they affect the Quadruple Aim? Why?

2. How would a divergent collaboration enable innovation in your organization and transform nursing practice with new workflows, models, products, or processes?

3. Identify three specific actions you can take to become innovative in your work. How will they impact your organization to evolve into an innovation engine?

REFERENCES

Ab Rahman, A., Abdul Hamid, U. K., & Chin, T. A. (2017). Emerging technologies with disruptive effects: A review. *PERINTIS eJournal, 7*(2), 111–128. Retrieved from https://perintis.org.my/ejournal/wp-content/uploads/2018/11/Paper-4-Vol.-7-No.-2-pp.-111-128.pdf

Adner, R., & Levinthal, D. A. (2002). The emergence of emerging technologies. *California Management Review, 45*(1), 50–66. doi:10.2307/41166153

Agarawal, S. (2018). *Helpsy Health: Personalized care planning platform and referral network.* Retrieved from https://www.medstartr.com/project/detail/1158

American Hospital Association. (n.d.). *About the AHA Center for Health Innovation.* Retrieved from https://www.aha.org/center/about-center-health-innovation

Bodenheimer, T., & Sinsky, C. (2014). From Triple to Quadruple Aim: Care of the patient requires care of the provider. *Annals of Family Medicine, 12*(6), 573–576. doi:10.1370/afm.1713

Bresnick, J. (2018a, June 1). *Broader availability of genetic testing a boon for precision care.* Retrieved from https://healthitanalytics.com/news/broader-availability-of-genetic-testing-a-boon-for-precision-care

Bresnick, J. (2018b, June 27). *Microsoft places bid in the AI gold rush with new healthcare team.* Retrieved from https://healthitanalytics.com/news/microsoft-places-bid-in-the-ai-gold-rush-with-new-healthcare-team

Browne, R. (2018, August 17). *Tech firms say A.I. can transform health care as we know it. Doctors think they should slow down.* Retrieved from https://www.cnbc.com/2018/08/17/healthcare-and-ai-doctors-warn-on-the-pace-of-technological-change.html

Carroll, W. (n.d.). *Hit the road! A guide for nursing innovation.* Retrieved from http://nurseevolution.com/hit-the-road-a-guide-for-nursing-innovation/

Castellanos, S. (2017, May 16). Why your pharmacy may be texting you. *Wall Street Journal.* Retrieved from https://www.wsj.com/articles/why-your-pharmacy-may-be-texting-you-1494986940

CB Insights. (2017, September 20). *Apple is going after the health care industry, starting with personal health data.* Retrieved from https://www.cbinsights.com/research/apple-health-care-strategy-apps-expert-research

Centers for Disease Control and Prevention. (2018). *Social Determinants of Health: Know what affects health—frequently asked questions.* Retrieved from https://www.cdc.gov/socialdeterminants/faqs/#faq1

Christensen, C. (2018). *Disruptive innovation—Key concepts.* Retrieved from http://www.claytonchristensen.com/key-concepts

Cianelli, R., Clipper, B., Freeman, R., Goldstein, J., & Wyatt, T. (2016). *The innovation road map: A guide for nurse leaders.* Retrieved from https://www.nursingworld.org/globalassets/ana/innovations-roadmap-english.pdf

Cleveland Clinic Innovations. (n.d.). *Our process.* Retrieved from https://innovations.clevelandclinic.org/Innovations/Our-Process-Overview.aspx

Correa-de-Araujo, R. (2017). Enhancing data access and utilization: Federal big data initiative and relevance to health disparities research. In C. W. Delaney, C. A. Weaver, J. J. Warren, T. R. Clancy, & R. L. Simpson (Eds.), *Big Data-enabled nursing: Education, research and practice* (p. 241). Cham, Switzerland: Springer Nature.

Daniel, G. W., Colvin, H. M., Silcox, C. E., McClellan, M. B., & Bryan, J. M. (Eds.). (2016). *The National Evaluation System for Health Technology (NEST): Priorities for effective early implementation*. Retrieved from https://healthpolicy.duke.edu/sites/default/files/atoms/files/NEST%20Priorities%20for%20Effective%20Early%20Implementation%20September%202016_0.pdf

Davidson, S., Weberg, D., Porter-O'Grady, T., & Malloch, K. (2017). *Leadership for evidence-based innovation in nursing and health professions*. Burlington, MA: Jones & Bartlett.

Day, G., & Schoemaker, P. (Eds.). (2000). *Wharton on managing emerging technologies*. New York, NY: John Wiley and Sons.

Dyer, J. H., Gregersen, H. B., & Christensen, C. M. (2011). *The Innovator's DNA: Mastering the five skills of disruptive innovators*. Boston, MA: Harvard Business Press.

The Economist. (2017). *Jeremy Corbyn, entrepreneur*. Retrieved from https://www.economist.com/britain/2017/06/15/jeremy-corbyn-entrepreneur

Emerging technologies. (n.d.). In *BusinessDictionary* online. Retrieved from http://www.businessdictionary.com/definition/emerging-technologies.html

Fast Company. (2018). *The world's most innovative companies 2018 honorees by sector*. Retrieved from https://www.fastcompany.com/most-innovative-companies/2018/sectors/health

Gartner Newsroom. (2017). *Gartner says by 2020, artificial intelligence will create more jobs than it eliminates*. Retrieved from https://www.gartner.com/en/newsroom/press-releases/2017-12-13-gartner-says-by-2020-artificial-intelligence-will-create-more-jobs-than-it-eliminates

Gaskell, A. (2017, June 19). The collaborative nature of healthcare innovation. *Forbes Magazine*. Retrieved from https://www.forbes.com/sites/adigaskell/2017/06/19/the-collaborative-nature-of-healthcare-innovation

Gershgorn, D. (2018, September 6). *If AI is going to be the world's doctor, it needs better textbooks*. Retrieved from https://qz.com/1367177/if-ai-is-going-to-be-the-worlds-doctor-it-needs-better-textbooks

Halaweh, M. (2013). Emerging technology: What is it? *Journal of Technology Management & Innovation, 8*(3), 108–115. doi:10.4067/S0718-27242013000400010

Healthcare Information and Management Systems Society. (2011). *Defining clinical transformation*. Retrieved from https://www.himss.org/news/defining-clinical-transformation

Healthcare Information and Management Systems Society. (n.d.-a). *About HIMSS*. Retrieved from https://www.himss.org/about-himss

Healthcare Information and Management Systems Society. (n.d.-b). *The HIMSS Innovation Center*. Retrieved from https://www.himssinnovationcenter.org

Helpsy Health. (2019a). *About us*. Retrieved from https://helpsyhealth.com/aboutus

Helpsy Health. (2019b). *Centers*. Retrieved from https://helpsyhealth.com/center

Holzman, S. B., Zenilman, A., & Shah, M. (2018). Advancing patient-centered care in tuberculosis management: A mixed-methods appraisal of video directly observed therapy. *Open Forum Infectious Diseases, 5*(4), ofy046. doi:10.1093/ofid/ofy046

Huynh, N. (2018, August 27). *How the "Big 4" tech companies are leading healthcare innovation*. Retrieved from https://healthcareweekly.com/how-the-big-4-tech-companies-are-leading-healthcare-innovation

Institute of Medicine. (2010). *The future of nursing: Leading change, advancing health*. Retrieved from http://books.nap.edu/openbook.php?record_id=12956&page=R1

The Joint Commission. (2016). *Quick safety: Issue 23—Implicit bias in health care*. Retrieved from https://www.jointcommission.org/assets/1/23/Quick_Safety_Issue_23_Apr_2016.pdf

Lehoux, P., Gauthier, P., Williams-Jones, B., Miller, F. A., Fishman, J. R., Hivon, M., & Vachon, P. (2014). Examining the ethical and social issues of health technology design through the public appraisal of prospective scenarios: A study protocol describing a multimedia-based deliberative method. *Implementation Science*, *9*, 81. doi:10.1186/1748-5908-9-81

Lovett, L. (2018, June 11). *Glooko launches diabetes analytics platform*. Retrieved from https://www.mobihealthnews.com/content/glooko-launches-diabetes-analytics-platform

Lucker, J., Hogan, S. K., & Sniderman, B. (2018, July 30). *Fooled by the hype—Is it the next big thing or merely a shiny new object?* Retrieved from https://www2.deloitte.com/content/dam/insights/us/articles/4437_fooled-by-the-hype/DI_fooled-by-the-hype.pdf

Macfarquhar, L. (2012, May 12). When giants fail: What business has learned from Clayton Christensen. *The New Yorker*. Retrieved from https://www.newyorker.com/magazine/2012/05/14/when-giants-fail

McGonigle, D., & Mastrian, K. (2017). *Nursing informatics and the foundation of knowledge* (4th ed., p. 111). Burlington, MA: Jones & Bartlett.

Millea, J., Green, I., & Putland, G. (2005). *Emerging technologies: A framework for thinking. Australian Capital Territory Department of Education and Training; Final report*. Retrieved from http://hdl.voced.edu.au/10707/54114

Mitchell, S. (2007). The import of uncertainty. *The Pluralist*, *2*(1), 58–71. Retrieved from http://www.jstor.org/stable/20708888

Muoio, D. (2018, May 18). *In-depth: Therapeutic VR in 2018 is no longer just a distraction (therapy)*. Retrieved from https://www.mobihealthnews.com/content/depth-therapeutic-vr-2018-no-longer-just-distraction-therapy

Nagle, L. M., & Yetman, L. (2009). Moving to a culture of nurse as knowledge worker and a new way of knowing in nursing. *Studies in Health Technology and Informatics*, *146*, 467–472. doi:10.3233/978-1-60750-024-7-467

National Academies of Sciences, Engineering, and Medicine. (2018). *Crossing the quality chasm: The IOM health care quality initiative*. Retrieved from http://www.nationalacademies.org/hmd/Global/News%20Announcements/Crossing-the-Quality-Chasm-The-IOM-Health-Care-Quality-Initiative.aspx

National Institutes of Health—U.S. National Library of Medicine. (2018, October 30). *What is direct-to-consumer genetic testing?* Retrieved from https://ghr.nlm.nih.gov/primer/dtcgenetictesting/directtoconsumer

O'Bryan, M. (2017). *Innovation: The most important and overused word in America*. Retrieved from https://www.wired.com/insights/2013/11/innovation-the-most-important-and-overused-word-in-america

Patient-Centered Primary Care Collaborative. (2018, August). *Advanced primary care: A key contributor to successful ACOS—PCPCC annual evidence report*. Retrieved from https://www.pcpcc.org/resource/evidence2018

Ready, T. (2017, June 15). *Data on social needs may redefine precision healthcare*. Retrieved from https://www.healthleadersmedia.com/clinical-care/data-social-needs-may-redefine-precision-healthcare

Rotolo, D., Hicks, D., & Martin, B. R. (2015). What is an emerging technology? *Research Policy*, *44*(10), 1827–1843. doi:10.1016/j.respol.2015.06.006

Simonite, T., (2018, May 11). The Trump administration plays catch-up on artificial intelligence. *Wired*. Retrieved from https://www.wired.com/story/trump-administration-plays-catch-up-artificial-intelligence/

Slabodkin, G. (2018, September 6). *AHA launches Center for Health Innovation to advance healthcare*. Retrieved from https://www.healthdatamanagement.com/news/aha-launches-center-for-health-innovation-to-advance-healthcare

Srinivasan, R. (2008). Sources, characteristics and effects of emerging technologies: Research opportunities in innovation. *Industrial Marketing Management, 37*, 633–640. doi:10.1016/j.indmarman.2007.12.003

Stahl, B. C. (2011). What does the future hold? A critical view of emerging information and communication technologies and their social consequences. In M. Chiasson, O. Henfridsson, H. Karsten, & J. I. DeGross (Eds.), *Researching the future in information systems* (pp. 59–76). Berlin, Germany: Springer.

Stoller, K. (2018). The world's largest tech companies 2018: Apple, Samsung take top spots again. *Forbes.* Retrieved from https://www.forbes.com/sites/kristinstoller/2018/06/06/worlds-largest-tech-companies-2018-global-2000/#28ce166b4de6

Stone, S. (2017, January 23). Why every company is a technology company. *Forbes.* Retrieved from https://www.forbes.com/sites/forbestechcouncil/2017/01/23/why-every-company-is-a-technology-company/#7b4086657aec

Sullivan, T. (2017, September 21). *Here's where hospitals are investing in innovation today.* Retrieved from https://www.healthcareitnews.com/news/heres-where-hospitals-are-investing-innovation-today

Sullivan, T. (2018, March 2). *HIMSS acquires Healthbox to get in the innovation consulting game.* Retrieved from https://www.healthcareitnews.com/news/himss-acquires-healthbox-get-innovation-consulting-game

U.S. Food and Drug Administration. (2018a). *FDA statement: Statement from FDA Commissioner Scott Gottlieb, M.D. and Jeff Shuren, M.D., Director of the Center for Devices and Radiological Health, on FDA's updates to Medical Device Safety Action Plan to enhance post-market safety.* Retrieved from https://www.fda.gov/NewsEvents/Newsroom/PressAnnouncements/ucm626286.htm

U.S. Food and Drug Administration. (2018b). *Medical Device Safety Action Plan: Protecting patients, promoting public health.* Retrieved from https://www.fda.gov/AboutFDA/CentersOffices/OfficeofMedicalProductsandTobacco/CDRH/CDRHReports/ucm604500.htm

Vera Whole Health. (2018). *Benefit strategy design: Solving an impossible task* [White Paper]. Retrieved from https://content.verawholehealth.com/benefit-strategy-design-solving-an-impossible-task

Vera Whole Health. (2019). *Methodology—Advanced primary care.* Retrieved from https://www.verawholehealth.com/advanced-primary-care

The White House. (2015, October 21). *Fact sheet: The White House releases new Strategy for American Innovation, announces areas of opportunity from self-driving cars to smart cities.* Retrieved from https://obamawhitehouse.archives.gov/the-press-office/2015/10/21/fact-sheet-white-house-releases-new-strategy-american-innovation

Wicklund, E. (2018, April 26). *mHealth program uses smartphones to monitor medication adherence.* Retrieved from https://mhealthintelligence.com/news/mhealth-program-uses-smartphones-to-monitor-medication-adherence

World Health Organization. (2018). *About social determinants of health.* Retrieved from http://www.who.int/social_determinants/sdh_definition/en

Zand, P. (2017). *Advancing innovation in health care.* Retrieved from https://www.hhnmag.com/articles/8601-advancing-innovation-in-health-care

ADDITIONAL RESOURCES

American Pharmacists Association. (2017, May 17). *CVS health pushing the boundaries of innovation.* Retrieved from https://www.pharmacist.com/article/cvs-health-pushing-boundaries-innovation

Grifantini, K. (2015). Incubating innovation: A standard model for nurturing new businesses, the incubator gains prominence in the world of biotech. *IEEE Pulse*, *6*(6), 27–31. doi:10.1109/MPUL.2015.2476542

Ready, T. (2017). *Data on social needs may redefine precision healthcare.* Retrieved from http://www.healthleadersmedia.com/quality/data-social-needs-may-redefine-precision-healthcare

2

Nursing Value and Big Data

WHENDE M. CARROLL

CHAPTER OBJECTIVES

- Define value-based care in the current healthcare landscape.
- Describe how nursing value directly impacts the Quadruple Aim.
- Understand Big Data characteristics and flow of end-to-end processing of Big Data.
- Comprehend the imperatives of data-driven emerging technology adoption and application in practice.

CONTENTS

INTRODUCTION

The equation of cost over quality equals value. In healthcare, this equation stands as new value-based care initiatives abound, where nursing can be at the forefront. The use of health information technology (IT) in practice impacts value. Where currently the cost of nursing care goes mostly unnoticed, the use of emerging technologies significantly impacts practice and adds value. Nurse informaticists and innovators add value to healthcare. Novel technologies used in clinical practice rely on core data to feed the health IT ecosystem for the development, use, and sustainment of emerging technologies. The reliance on vast amounts of data, known as Big Data, as a technological imperative in health IT lies in the understanding of what data are, their impact on the life cycle of emerging technologies, and benefit to nursing in advancing the profession through improving value-based care and serving the **Quadruple Aim**.

VALUE-BASED CARE

The definition of **value-based care** is cost over quality, with the "value" in value-based healthcare stemming from measuring health outcomes against the cost of delivering outcomes (New England Journal of Medicine [NEJM], 2017). Today, healthcare organizations and providers look to improve quality of care for patients and expect adequate reimbursement in return. Although fee-for-service began moving to pay-for-performance more than two decades ago, the impetus of the need for value-based care was the inception of the Patient Protection and Affordable Care Act (ACA) put into legislation in 2010. The set of laws aim to increase access to care of the over 75,000 underinsured or uninsured Americans and decrease healthcare costs while improving quality of healthcare delivery with programs abounding with new rules for reimbursement and costs savings led by government entities (Salmond & Forrester, 2016). The requirements for the Centers for Medicaid and Medicare services have changed how health-care organizations and providers receive payment for patient care delivery for Medicare patients (Centers for Medicare and Medicaid Services [CMS], 2018). Subsequently, value-based care approaches, programs, and models (Salmond & Echevarria, 2017) have evolved from provider reimbursements for volume for care provided to pay for performance based on payments that return quality patient outcomes (Miller, 2009).

Value-based care models establish payments grounded in care quality out-comes, including value-based purchasing, and bundled care estimates costs and determines payments through the care quality provided throughout the continuum of patient care (NEJM, 2017). Also, the value-based model of Accountable Care Organizations (ACOs) can realize savings by using population health models for more efficient and less costly care. The move to these programs and models serves to better manage care through a patient's complete episode of care to provide value (BHM Marketing, 2016). The steps toward value-based care have required the integration of healthcare technology to make it possible; healthcare organizations are incentivized to provide improved management of patients, decreased cost, and improved patient experience—all equating to value—for reimbursement (CMS, 2018; see Table 2.1).

Table 2.1 Value-Based Care Programs and Models

Value-based purchasing	Healthcare organization pays for performance for Medicare patients • Reimbursement based on quality outcomes, including patient satisfaction, efficiency, care coordination, and safety • Aligns quality of care incentives across providers and payers
Bundled care payments	Targeted at decreasing costs by reducing unnecessary services for a surgery or episode of care based on diagnosis • Providers and payers mutually decide on episodic care cost. • Economic risk is assumed by providers and reimbursements, or savings, are shared among providers who manage patients most efficiently with the best outcomes.
Accountable Care Organizations	Aimed at improved care coordination, efficiency, and promotion of preventative service to maximize wellness • Networks of health organizations and providers that take collective accountability for the cost and quality of care for specific cohorts of patients over time • Paid on a fee-for-service plan with additional incentives to participate in shared savings percentage of any realized savings
Population health	Focused on people with specific conditions (i.e., diabetes, COPD, maternal care) • A paradigm shift that aligns care of a particular diagnosis or disease through providing care based on risk stratification and measuring outcomes of patient cohorts over time • Reimbursement is dependent on the cost associated with the full management of the population having a condition.
PCMH	Focused on the collective delivery of higher quality, cost-effective primary care deemed essential for patients with chronic health conditions • Shared elements include shared common elements including *comprehensive, patient-centered, coordinated, accessible care* across the continuum of patient care. • Puts provider emphasis on safety and quality by using clinical decision support tools, shared decision-making, evidence-based care, and performance indicators to measure patients and PCMH outcomes

COPD, chronic obstructive pulmonary disease; PCMH, patient-centered medical home.

These revolutionary approaches, programs, and models increase value and service to meet the Quadruple Aim in healthcare, and achieving this imperative requires IT. CMS requires healthcare organizations and providers to show how technology, particularly electronic health records (EHRs), is transmitting information electronically to provide the benefits of patients' medication management, preventative care services, and clinical engagement and experience, the full spectrum of patients' quality in care delivery (Office of the National Coordinator for Health Information Technology, 2008). To meet these needs, healthcare IT as a business evolves with innovation as the major part of serving the Quadruple Aim and providing value in healthcare. The use of health IT innovation is impacting value-based care by supporting the underpinnings and mechanisms, and measuring the success, of new quality of care models, for example, furthering the efforts of the creation of national population health and public and community health initiatives with healthcare data analytics at the core (Healthcare Information and Management Systems Society, 2017).

NURSES IMPACT VALUE-BASED CARE

As healthcare systems ease into reimbursement for the value-based care environment and provide safety and quality outcomes at a lower cost, nursing will have a significant impact on the success of these efforts and will be the most altered by the evolution to value-based care. To begin with, there are two nursing imperatives to quantify value-based nursing care—first, articulating the nursing product and prices for the provided services; and second, determining the economic value of nursing care to the healthcare organization (Caspers & Pickard, 2013). To meet the requirements of value-based care approaches and programs, care transformation will entail a concerted effort by nurses to become savvier to the disruption of healthcare business models and be at the forefront to utilize technology for making crucial changes in patient safety, quality, and patient experience.

Health organization labor represents approximately 68% of all inpatient operational cost, with all nursing labor cost representing about 30%, equating to nearly a quarter trillion dollars ($216.7 billion) per year for inpatient nursing care (Welton, 2015). The nursing workforce represents the largest segment of the healthcare workforce with more than 3 million licensed nurses (U.S. Department of Health and Human Services, 2014). Nursing is once again the most respected profession. For the 17th consecutive year, Americans' ratings of the honesty and ethical standards of 22 occupations find nurses at the top of the Gallup Poll, which analyzes occupations as an economic stimulus factor. More than four in five (84%) Americans describe nurses' ethics as "very high" or "high" (Brenan, 2018). With these truths, the shift to value-based care models and the efforts needed for initiatives to help providers and healthcare organizations improve management of populations, reduce costs, and improve patient satisfaction relies heavily on nursing. Evolving patient care for safety, enhanced efficiency, providing evidence-based connected care and patient engagement, and developing learning healthcare organizations and new care models that support workflows influencing these factors are central to nursing care delivery. If nurses are crucial to changing the clinical processes that impact value-based care, the tangible and intangible elements that institute value are essential to capture and measure (Welton & Harper, 2015).

In value-based models, the impact of nursing care relative to value remains largely invisible (Delaney, Weaver, Warren, Clancy, & Simpson, 2017). To date, the provision of nursing care has been deemed intangible versus tangible (Rutherford, 2008) in the equation and outcomes of direct payment and reimbursement for patient care in the same way as healthcare organizations and providers. Pappas (2013) defines "nursing value" as the function of outcomes divided by costs. Nursing care delivery drives value, and nurses have a direct and intimate influence on the quality, safety, and costs of patient-centered care. In describing nursing value as the function of outcomes divided by costs, there is a need to better define the measures and analytics for patient-level costs and outcomes of nursing care (Pappas, 2013). One way purveyors of value-based care can identify and influence nursing care delivery as a driver in the pay for value environment is through the use of data, advanced analytics, and emerging technologies (Carroll & Hofmeister, 2018). The involvement of nursing in the entire life cycle, including conception, development, implementation, use, sustainment, and enhancement, will raise the impact of value-based care as it is dependent on nursing as a catalyst of innovation and as an adopter of emerging technology.

The Importance of Nursing Value in New Models of Care

Healthcare organizations that ignore the costs associated with patient–nurse time would be increasingly disadvantaged with value-based payment changes (Pappas & Welton, 2015). Staffing, nursing-sensitive indicators, and financial outcomes have critical relationships to value-based programs, for both economic health and patient outcomes (Pappas, Davidson, Woodard, Davis, & Welton, 2015).

For the recognition of nurses' worth in value-based care, the assets of nursing value to the profession at large first need to be identified. Quantification of these drivers to the business model of healthcare, concerning profitability, is imperative to this. **Nurse value drivers** are operational factors in value creation, with these valuable assets being both tangible and intangible (Rutherford, 2010). Value drivers in value-based care include the more straightforward aspects of nursing knowledge, revenue, efficiencies, and patient care outcomes. Trust, caring, and intuition also need to be taken into account as drivers of value, although they are less easy to calculate (Rutherford, 2010). These drivers align objectives, harmonize professional goals, guide industry investment, and identify financial and operational factors (see Figure 2.1).

Two additional value drivers are nurse intellectual capital and economic worth, the unique assets that impact value-based care models, particularly the needs to

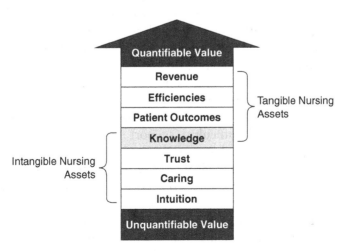

Figure 2.1 Nursing value drivers assets scale.

provide quality outcomes while reducing costs. This is imperative to meeting the goals of value-based care for provider groups and healthcare organizations to improve reimbursement and cost savings. Intellectual capital is the combination of collective knowledge in an organization or society. It is an intangible asset encompassing a group of individuals possessing knowledge about the processes, customers, and other information to contribute to improved business performance or profits. Management of these assets is the process of effectively utilizing the knowledge to gain a competitive advantage for the organization. Knowledge in healthcare organizations facilitates decision-making while delivering patient care and contributes to gaining new knowledge and stimulating innovation (Covell & Sidani, 2013); this improves performance and has direct links to improved business performance and quality patient care (Aiken et al., 2011). A tangible asset is nurse economic value demonstrated by cost-related services. The ability to gain payment for services is strongly linked to the strength of the nursing profession to define the value of its service. Valuation as an economic term is used to determine worth or value, and, as a field or endeavor, involves financial valuing of a company's resources. Financial analyses must look at both quantitative and qualitative aspects of the business through valuation studies. These provide a more precise depiction of the business of healthcare's resources, including the identification of both tangible and intangible assets that represent value (Rutherford, 2008). To prove nurses' worth and what they bring to value-based care, these need to be quantified, and nurses acknowledged as the vital force that keeps patients safe, delivers high-quality care, directly lowers costs, implores patient-centered care to improve patient experience and satisfaction—which are all needed for value-based programs to succeed.

Measuring Nursing Value

With nurses at the forefront to accomplish the goals of value-based programs, technology will play a significant role. In healthcare settings, nursing care is hidden among procedure codes for fee-for-service and emerging value-based reimbursement. The variation in nursing resources provided to each patient is virtually unknown, and there is no alignment among nursing direct-care time and costs, billing for nursing services, and payment for care. This will become increasingly problematic as payers, such as CMS, move toward value-based payment models and they will have greater accountability to improve outcomes of care and share costs (Welton, 2010; Welton & Harper, 2015).

The ability to identify the impact of best nursing practices and the optimum level of nursing care will be essential factors in ascertaining value within a value-based healthcare system. Unfortunately, nursing is absent from these discussions, making it difficult to support new payment models when nursing costs and intensity are unknown (Welton, 2010). The addition of new nursing-specific data linked to individual patients within the costing and billing system will allow improved analysis of nursing care and will require treating nursing care in a more businesslike manner consistent with emerging value-based frameworks (Welton, 2010). The growing focus on nursing care value involves the development of tangible assets and measurable aspects of nursing care such as scheduling and staffing unique identifier data to link nurses directly to individual patients.

Historically this has been challenging to achieve as most clinical and operational records were paper-based, and the cost to use these records for such purposes did not outweigh the benefits (Finkler, 2008).

The implementation of EHRs solves this problem, and the current focus is on identifying and extracting relevant patient care data from the EHR and development of new analytic models to measure nursing care delivery (Welton & Harper, 2015). Using a rich multidisciplinary data source, it will be possible to measure team interaction, continuity of care, and nursing outcomes across multiple healthcare settings, and where efforts to define nursing care value were hindered by a lack of available data, new information from EHRs now provides an opportunity to measure nursing care in ways that have not been possible (Welton & Harper, 2015).

Understanding the reasons behind the lack of cost-related nurse data as well as realizing the need to accumulate cost data related to nursing services can stimulate efforts. Data documenting both the tangible and intangible assets of nursing service are needed to communicate its value fully. Valuation initiatives can build information that will substantiate the community's demand for adequate investment in nursing (Rutherford, 2010). Nursing value can be hard to measure as intangible assets and is generally unquantifiable. To date, point-of-care documentation data have made it possible to quantify what nursing does clinically and administratively. The focus now turns to the EHR, enterprise resource planning, and other health IT systems to measure nursing value. With the emergence of large data sets, nurses now have not only the opportunity to be a part of the conversation about value-based care but also become pioneers in defining value through the advanced use of technology with and beyond the EHR (Case Study 2.1).

New Nurse Roles Support Value and Emerging Technology

As evidenced by Case Study 2.1, nurses have begun to take the lead in measuring the value of nursing using technology as the pay-for-quality landscape grows. The emergence of new roles for transforming care using data and analytics is shifting to support the outcomes of value-based care. Nurses are well-positioned to contribute to and lead the transformative changes that are occurring in healthcare by being fully engaged members of the interprofessional team through the movement from episodic, provider-based, fee-for-service care to team-based, patient-centered care across the continuum that uses new and enhanced sets of knowledge, skills, and attitudes to provide continuous, cost-effective, and quality care (Salmond & Echevarria, 2017).

Nurse informaticists, innovators, entrepreneurs, and data scientists are coming to the forefront to ignite these essential changes in value-based care focused on patient outcomes (see Table 2.2). Nurses, in these unique and developing specialties, have a significant impact on value-based programs and models and add relevancy and potency and ways to quantify the intangible assets of the value brought to the profession. They are increasingly the conceptualizers, inventors, champions, investors, and peddlers of products, services, and new processes that support the implementation and adoption of emerging technologies. Collectively, these evolving specialists have the experience and expertise to use data to

CASE STUDY 2.1

TOWARD SHARABLE AND COMPARABLE NURSE DATA: NURSING KNOWLEDGE BIG DATA SCIENCE INITIATIVE

The 'data-rich, knowledge-poor' state of healthcare (Westra et al., 2015), in the era that Big Data are upon us with the dawning of the EHR, provides nurse data scientists the means for the discovery of knowledge value through the use of sharable and comparable nurse-sensitive data, and create knowledge engineering through the use of advanced computational methods to develop knowledge value (Westra et al., 2015). A guided effort to have nurses fully realize the power of Big Data was established in 2013 as a collaborative where nurse leaders gathered to create a National Action Plan to demonstrate nurse value through data derived from EHRs and other health IT systems, by convening at the University of Minnesota. The first meeting, consisting of nearly 30 participants, has since evolved into 150+ annual conferences of national nurse leaders who are now members of 11 workgroups that aim to create a culture of data specific to demonstrating nursing value through data, now known as the *Nursing Knowledge: Big Data Science (KNBDS) Conference.*

The NKBDS initiative's core mission across these 6 years has been to develop a roadmap for achieving sharable and comparable nurse-sensitive data, ensuring the timely adoption of Big Data methodologies across all of nursing's domains, and creating a vision of better health outcomes for individuals, families, and communities empowered by the standardization and integration of the information nurses gather in EHRs and other information systems (University of Minnesota School of Nursing [UMNSON], 2019). Nurses committed to advancing the discovery of nursing knowledge achieve health improvements and efficiencies that come from guaranteeing that nursing data captured in EHRs and other sources are available in sharable and comparable formats to support useful, actionable insights by clinicians, researchers, policy makers, and patients.

The 2018 workgroup reports demonstrate the considerable evolution that has occurred over these past 6 years, the significant body of work completed, and breadth of accomplishments achieved from nationally known nurse participants from healthcare, standards, and nursing organizations, health IT vendors, nursing academia, and nurse researchers and entrepreneurs (NKBDS Conference, 2018). The growth of the initiative and Action Plans now developed by health IT nurses at this conference has expanded to 11 distinct groups that support nursing education, policy, mobile health, and clinical data analytics, among others. The 2018 workgroups and purpose include (NKBDS Conference, 2018):

CARE COORDINATION

Identify nursing implications related to Big Data associated with care coordination across the healthcare continuum.

(continued)

CASE STUDY 2.1 (*continued*)

CLINICAL DATA ANALYTICS

Demonstrate the value of sharable and comparable nurse-sensitive data to enhance care delivery and translational research for transforming healthcare and improving patient safety and quality.

CONTEXT OF CARE

Capture nursing Big Data in the Nursing Management Minimum Data Set (NMMDS), the Nursing Minimum Data Set (NMDS), and the Nursing Knowledge: Big Data Science Conference Nursing Value Data Set (NVDS) to increase nurse data usability; provide patient, family, and community-centric data; and reinforce data generated by nurses, about nurses, and nursing care.

EDUCATION

Strengthen informatics education at the graduate and specialty levels and the ability of educators who teach informatics to achieve the outcomes of nursing data through the work of nurses at the point of care.

ENCODING AND MODELING

Develop and disseminate standard nursing care terms for EHR nursing assessments and incorporate them into a framework and repository for dissemination.

ENGAGE AND EQUIP ALL NURSES IN HEALTH IT POLICY

Equip nurses with knowledge and tools, and the means to engage them as expert advocates for health IT policy efforts essential to nursing.

MOBILE HEALTH FOR NURSING

Explore the use of mobile health tools and data by nurses including both nursing-generated data and patient-generated data to identify and support activities and resources to address unmet needs and create opportunities to use mobile health data within nursing workflows.

NURSING VALUE

Measure the value of nursing care as well as the contribution of individual nurses to clinical outcomes and cost, and develop Big Data techniques for secondary data

(continued)

CASE STUDY 2.1 (*continued*)

analysis providing metrics to monitor quality, costs, performance, effectiveness, and efficiency of nursing care.

SOCIAL DETERMINANTS OF HEALTH

Support the inclusion, interoperability, and data exchange of **Social Determinants of Health** (SDoH) data in EHRs, personal and mobile health tools, and community and public health portals across care settings, with the intent to empower nurses to use SDoH data as context for planning care and develop a roadmap to engage nurses in improving population health through large-scale adoption of health determinants.

STREAMLINING/TRANSFORMING DOCUMENTATION

Explore ways to decrease the documentation burden and serve up the information already in the EHR at the right time in the workflow to support evidence-based and personalized care by fast-tracking the integration of best clinical knowledge into care decisions (Smith, Saunders, Stuckhardt, & McGinnis, 2013).

E-REPOSITORY

Develop and implement an assets store designed to collect nursing informatics best evidence, including documents, surveys, instruments, and algorithms, to catalogue and disseminate the work completed by the workgroups for all nurses to leverage and create a data culture and support knowledge engineering.

This evolution toward a culture of data that is inclusive, less burdensome, sharable, and comparable demonstrates nursing value by the legions of nurses joining this conference and workgroups each summer at the University of Minnesota. This enormous effort, guided by Big Data and nursing works to include environmental, geographical, and behavioral information, is an increasing source of insights and evidence produced by data that aims to prevent, diagnose, treat, and evaluate health conditions. The effort to disrupt healthcare and further nurses' understanding of data for advancing the health of individuals, families, communities, and populations is the mission of the movement (UMNSON, 2019).

disseminate information, knowledge, and wisdom through the use of health IT. By doing this, nurses are new authorities in information management, including knowledge acquisition and distribution. As nursing knowledge doubles every 6 years, nurses are no longer the keepers of knowledge, but instead have become the masters of collecting and sharing that knowledge with others within and outside nursing (Huston, 2013) by taking the lead as the creators of what's next in nursing and healthcare (see Table 2.2).

Table 2.2 New Nurse Roles Using Technology to Transform Care Delivery

Nursing Role	Functions
Informatics specialists	Integrators of nursing science who work with multiple analytical sciences to identify, manage, and communicate data, information, and knowledge in nursing practice to support decision-making in all roles and settings to achieve desired outcomes for nurses, consumers, patients, interprofessional teams, and other stakeholders (American Nurses Association, 2015).
Innovators	Visionary change agents who encompass the characteristics of divergent thinking, risk-taking, failure tolerance, agility, flexibility, autonomy, and freedom to build a culture of novel thought with the intentional process of providing practical action and support of the attempts to introduce new and improved processes that disrupt current philosophies and rules governing healthcare reimbursement, access, delivery systems, and nursing education (Cianelli, Clipper, Freeman, Goldstein, & Wyatt, 2016).
Entrepreneurs	Experts who use nurse training, knowledge, and expertise to conventionalize and develop businesses within the healthcare industry through the use of creativity, commercial systems, problem-solving, and investing strategies to advance clinical applications for healthcare providers and patients focused on novel healthcare trends, procedures, practices, and the application of new and existing health information technology (Nurse Theory, 2018).
Data scientists	Advancers of nursing science who work with multiple sources of large data sets to extract information for testable explanations and predictions, develop and maintain a culture that embraces scholarly inquisitiveness, and advocate for the commitment of evidence-based knowledge, its application to practice and innovation, and conduct original research (Brant, 2015; Dhar, 2013).

With healthcare and technology moving at the speed of sound, nurses in these roles stay abreast of emerging trends, identify health systems and industry problems, and find ways to solve them, understanding that data and advanced analytics are at the core. With the industry focused on outcomes, these nurses transform care that spans the continuum, engages patients, and promotes connectivity in siloed systems. The emerging roles of nurse technologists, innovators, entrepreneurs, and nurse data scientists collectively harness the power of Big Data to disrupt the healthcare business models and add worth to new value-driven, evidence-based care delivery services, models, and processes to serve the Quadruple Aim.

BIG DATA

Data feed emerging technologies such as The Internet of Things, Artificial Intelligence, Predictive Analytics, Natural Language Processing, Virtual and Augmented Reality, Genomics, and Blockchain. Big Data at large is a buzzword used to describe the massive amounts of data that have flooded multiple business industries in the last few decades due to the increased use of computers. With each incidence and use on a computer of any size, data are generated and require storage. **Big Data** was initially described in 1997 by scientists at the National Aeronautics and Space Administration (NASA) as a problem. Computer graphics could not hold the amount of data needed for informative visualization. The term was coined as a challenge for computer systems as data sets became so large that they taxed the capacity of core memory stores on local disks, creating the need to acquire more resources, such as storage, to manage it (Cox & Ellsworth, 1997). Many definitions have followed, with a 2011 McKinsey report defining "Big Data" as "datasets whose size is beyond the ability of typical database software tools to capture, store, manage, and analyze" (Manyika et al., 2011, p. 1). The healthcare industry was cited as a domain that nets value from Big Data; however, one is challenged due to the vast amounts of information and storage needed to manage and manipulate it (Manyika et al., 2011).

Big Data in Healthcare

In healthcare, nurses generate a massive amount of data. Data are discrete objective entities whose interpretation and synthesis provide valuable information and knowledge. When digitally translated, they convey knowledge and further wisdom for actionable use in context (McGonigle & Mastrian, 2017). With the onslaught of clinical digitization, charting of patient care, using mobile health devices, integrating telecommunication equipment, and inputting information for administrative purposes has added to the influx of healthcare data. The healthcare industry produces up to 30% of the world's stored data, and a single patient typically generates close to 80 MB each year in imaging and EHR data. This tsunami of data has clear clinical, financial, and operational value with such data enabling more than $300 billion annually in reduced healthcare costs (Huesch & Mosher, 2017). While a seemingly daunting task, we are in an age where storage, management, and visualization are no longer challenging and in fact provide the opportunity to harness the power of Big Data to make actionable decisions to improve care quality and outcomes, promote system efficiencies, decrease variation in care, and improve clinical decision support systems.

DATA SOURCES

Sources of Big Data represent its vastness that is created every day from daily clinical and administrative workflows. Information and knowledge building is completed using the nursing process, including data generated from physical and functional assessments, condition diagnosis, care planning, carrying out interventions, and subsequent evaluation of patient progress and outcomes. This is true in all care environments, including data amassed from encounters in prescreening clinics, hospital units, outpatient clinics, virtual care, rehabilitation, long-term care through hospice, or patients moving back into the community. Two of the most significant opportunities for utilizing Big Data are in pre-hospital and

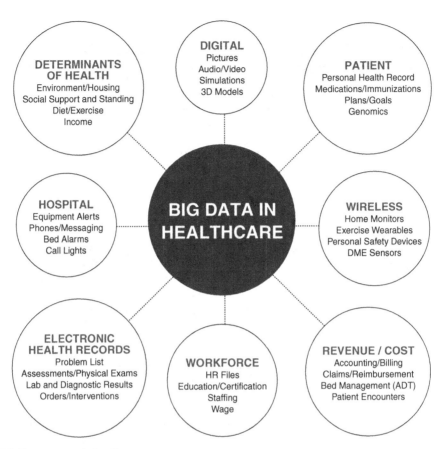

Figure 2.2 Data sources in healthcare.

ADT, admission, discharge, and transfer; DME, durable medical equipment; HR, human resources.

post-inpatient transitional care to connect all care delivery and administrative processes throughout the patient continuum. In addition, nurse workforce data can be used to demonstrate the value of nurses in the fee-for-service to pay-for-performance environment (Welton & Harper, 2015). See Figure 2.2 for Big Data sources (Welton & Harper, 2016). Within these sources, the challenge is to discretely and consistently collect SDoH data, and assure that the data sources used to create data sets represent all populations and are free of bias.

DATA CHARACTERISTICS

The Big Data generated daily in all industries has key features, known widely as the "Vs" (Grimes, 2013). Industry leaders and those associated with the research of Big Data name anywhere from 3 to 42 multidimensional Vs of Big Data and data science (Shafer, 2017). These terms explain Big Data's elements of enormity, function, diversity, performance, and usability. The ten essential **Vs of Big Data** to understand are (a) three fundamental features, the basic characteristics of all Big Data; (b) four intrinsic/structural, more capricious, sophisticated features; and (c) three crucial features, critical for outcomes and applications where Big Data are used (see Table 2.3) that relate to the composite whole, when data are stored, manipulated, and presented, and when applied, the benefits they bring to new business models, services, and processes.

Table 2.3 The 10 Vs of Big Data in Healthcare

Fundamental	
Volume	The enormous amount of data produced by hospital and healthcare workers each day. Example: EHR, enterprise resource planning, mobile health devices
Variety	The diversity of data types and data sources. Example: Patient claims, diagnosis and medication history, lab and radiology results
Velocity	Healthcare generates approximately 8 petabytes (PB) per year (Donovan, 2019)
Intrinsic/Structural	
Variability	The multiple sources and inconsistencies of data due to their disparate sources. Example: Data pulled from multiple health claims databases with varying configurations
Veracity	The data source reliability, its context, and how useful it is to the analysis based on it. Example: Incomplete or biased data causing poor performance of disease prediction
Volatility	The freshness of the data and their ongoing applicability to an analysis. Example: Old data in a laboratory database causing poor performance due to irrelevance
Vulnerability	The insecurity of the data, their sources, and the ability to be infringed and breached. Example: A healthcare insurer hack with 18,000,000 personal identification data stolen
Crucial	
Validity	The extent to how accurate and correct the data are for their intended use. Example: Missing demographic fields in ADT systems, multiple patient identifiers
Visualization	The structured presentation of processed data. Example: Charts, graphs, and dashboards representing hospital-acquired infection rates
Value	The benefits of the data for users. Example: Clinical decision support, predicting chronic illness, precise radiology results

ADT, admission, discharge, and transfer.
Source: Bresnick, J. (2017, June 5). *Understanding the many V's of healthcare Big Data analytics.* Retrieved from https://healthitanalytics.com/news/understanding-the-many-vs-of-healthcare-big-data-analytics; Firican, G. (2017, February 18). *The 10 Vs of Big Data.* Retrieved from https://tdwi.org/Articles/2017/02/08/10-Vs-of-Big-Data.aspx?Page=2

DATA CLASSIFICATION

Five main components commence the classification of Big Data (Figure 2.3). The elements considered are data sources, content format, data stores, data staging, and data processing (Mohanty, Bhuyan, & Chenthati, 2015). The sources generating data could be EHR, billing transactions, bed sensors, and Internet of Things-based medical devices. The content format of the data sources can be structured, unstructured, or semi-structured, which speaks to the data characteristic of variability. Data stores—structured places from where data are generated—include document- or column-oriented text and spreadsheets and data from graphic visualizations and those keyed into a machine, such as the EHR. Data staging speaks to the preprocessing of data that is required for management to prepare for information extraction, while data processing represents the necessary sequential approach to process Big Data (Mohanty et al., 2015). Big Data characteristics overarch these elements of classification and organize the data components, underscoring their complexity and reliance on resources to process data efficiently and effectively.

DATA PROCESSING

In healthcare and in all industries, there is a high-level approach to moving from data acquisition to actionable insights. Processing Big Data requires sequential steps that move from storage through output and prepares the data to be presented visually. Figure 2.4 outlines broad stages of data processing, including input, processing, and outputs with storage of data as the beginning and endpoint.

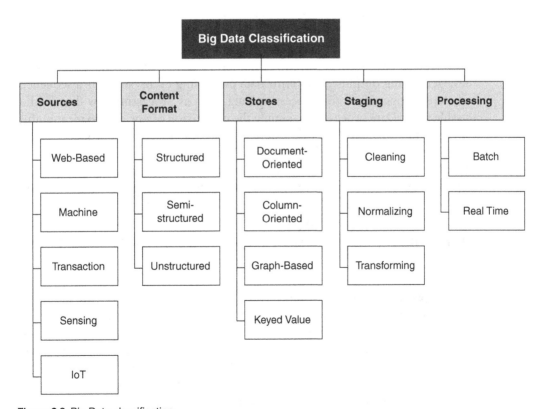

Figure 2.3 Big Data classification.

IoT, internet of things.

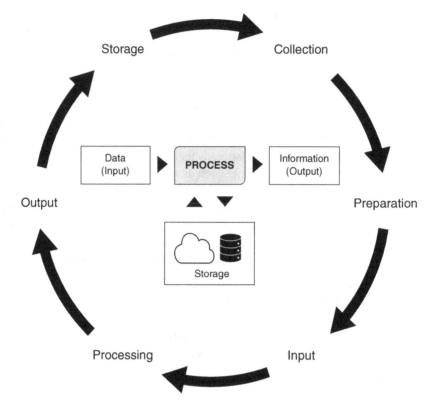

Figure 2.4 Big Data processing cycle.

They require substages of the larger process also outlined in the figure (Planning Tank, n.d.-b). Scientific data require numerous computations and usually need fast-generating outputs. The term "data processing cycle" suggests a sequence of steps or operations for processing data, such as processing raw data to the usable form. Data processing is simply the conversion of raw data to meaningful information through a process, where they are manipulated to produce results that lead to a resolution of a problem or improvement in an existing situation. Similar to a production process, it follows a cycle where inputs (raw data) are fed to a process (computer systems, software, etc.) to produce output (information and insights; Planning Tank, n.d.-a). Computer systems carry out a series of operations on the data to present, interpret, or obtain information. Useful output is presented in various appropriate formats, including reports and graphic visualizations.

DATA QUALITY

Just as patient care requires impeccable quality in execution for the best outcomes, so does Big Data for the correct outputs. Data quality is imperative for preparation of Big Data for processing and the accuracy of outputs (Arthofer & Girardi, 2017). There are five common Big Data quality domains—accuracy, completeness, consistency, credibility, and timeliness (Feder, 2018). Data accuracy is the overall truthfulness of the data. Techniques to evaluate data accuracy include comparing variables within the database or data set, known as internal validity; comparing variables with other external sources (external validity);

or comparing variables through data triangulation, the verification between multiple data sources, adding integrity to the findings. Data completeness is context driven and comprises the degree and type of missing values within a database or secondary data set. Data consistency pertains to the trustworthiness of the data at the needed level of detail for data manipulation, within and across databases and data sets; it requires careful selection of data sources and variables before data retrieval. Data credibility is the overall plausibility or reliability of the data in which data recognition is credible. Credibility can be predisposed by validation of the data from primary data sources and alignment of data with current knowledge and user-perceived reality. Although data credibility may appear similar to data accuracy, credibility relies on trustworthiness and the belief that the data reinforce a party's assumption of the environment (Feder, 2018). Data timeliness refers to the recency of data if data are inputted within a reasonable period from the sanctioned event, the overall age of the data, and relevancy of the data compared with current knowledge. For all data quality domains, data inaccuracies and incomplete data can result from significant postponements between data input and events. Furthermore, old data may reflect characteristics not necessarily generalizable to contemporary populations (Feder, 2018).

DATA VISUALIZATION

Data visualizations represent the outcomes of Big Data manipulation in the data-rich healthcare industry to guide decision-making in clinical or administrative practices. They act as the distribution structure that leads to interpretations of Big Data outputs. Data representations should conclusively tell robust stories of what is happening within the data—either quantitatively or qualitatively—and enable focused analysis of the data and information generation and sharing. Visualizations must be designed to work effectively with data quality (described in the "Data Quality" section) and should highlight deficiencies in the underlying data to users to consider as part of their analysis (Gotz & Borland, 2016). The fields of cognitive science and cognitive psychology have recognized that the human primary visual cortex is more effective and efficient at comparing variables, identifying patterns, and distinguishing relationships with shapes and colors than with numbers; therefore, data visualization is a desirable strategy for use in exploring large nursing data sets (Monsen et al., 2015). Various types of data visualization techniques exist to show different data analyses and must be carefully chosen to represent outcomes of data evaluations, including assessing part to whole relationships, determining changes over time, geospatial mapping, analyzing associations, and comparing categories (see Figure 2.5). Today, we use these visual representatives through leveraging computer science, statistics, and clinical expertise for visualization development and interpretation and human visual perception to identify salient, or apparent, distributions, patterns, or relationships in the Big Data (Gintautas, Kurasova, & Žilinskas, 2013). It is critical to align the purpose of the data project, transformation, and representation methods and make informed decisions based on sound visualization principles, to make visualizations effective (Monsen et al., 2015; Case Study 2.2).

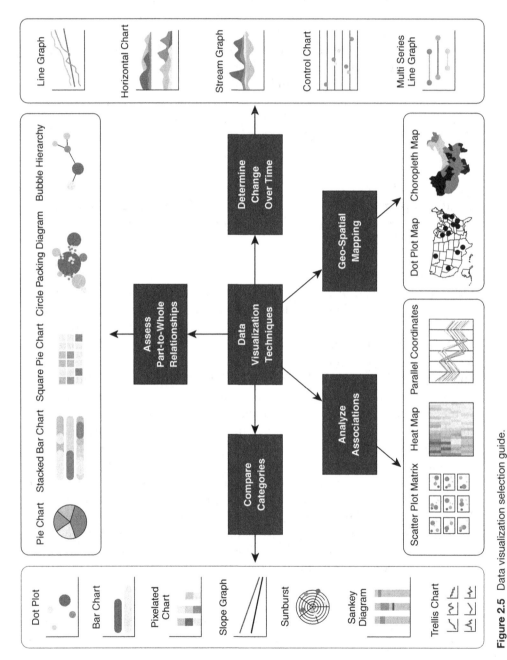

Figure 2.5 Data visualization selection guide.

Source: With permission from Monsen, K. A., Peterson, J. J., Mathiason, M. A., Kim, E., Lee, S., Chi, C.-L., & Pieczkiewicz, D. S. (2015). Data visualization techniques to showcase nursing care quality. *CIN—Computers Informatics Nursing, 33*(10), 417–426. doi:10.1097/CIN.0000000000000190

CASE STUDY 2.2

MAKING HEALTH DATA VISIBLE: FLORENCE NIGHTINGALE, A PIONEER OF DATA VISUALIZATION

Florence Nightingale, the "Lady With the Lamp," referring to her nighttime care to patients, is now widely considered to be the creator of epidemiology and modern nursing (Zaugg, Marchese, & Keller, n.d.). Arguably her most significant accomplishments, along with her work in public health and influencing current evidence-based practice, research, theory, and epidemiology, was studying and highlighting high mortality rates and preventable deaths of soldiers during the Crimean War of 1954 to 1956 where she served as a nurse leader and educator (Kopf, 1916).

When Florence Nightingale arrived in Crimea, there was no accurate count of the number of dead soldiers. To remedy this, Nightingale created forms and sent them to contacts throughout posts in Crimea to help document how many soldiers died and from what causes (Webb, 2010). She developed methods to track vital statistics and created universal paper forms to collect more precise patient medical information—procedures that are now commonplace and essential components of medical care, which "literally revolutionized hospital data collection" (Barbara Dossey as cited in Webb, 2010, "The Crimean War").

Armed with mathematics skills and a desire for understanding accurate counts of soldier deployments and deaths to measure outcomes and standardize practice, she manually counted the soldier's deaths in their hospital barracks. Throughout her data collection, Nightingale collaborated closely with well-known medical statisticians and used graphics to display her data to give the value-rich context, realizing early on that officials would likely ignore numbers without an attention-getting picture. Through her data collection, Nightingale discovered unknown patterns of infection and deaths—causes leading her to introduce sanitary measures, life-saving interventions implemented by physicians and nurses for soldiers that resulted in a decrease in mortality by 91% in 2 years (Lewi, 2006).

After returning from the war, Florence Nightingale presented her Crimea findings with the intention to convey the mortality rates and causes to the Sanitary Commission in Britain to improve practice, which proved to be very successful (Webb, 2010). This led her to very effectively use an early data visualization of the polar area diagram (see Figure 2.6), now referred to as the Rose Chart or "coxcomb" (Lewi, 2006), to visually communicate her findings.

The landmark data visualization is the well-known coxcomb graph, a precursor to the modern-day pie chart. The figure shows the stunning baseline mortality data from the Crimean War. The light gray wedges show the deaths from preventable diseases; the dark gray wedges show deaths from war wounds; and the blue wedges show deaths from all other causes. The circle divides the data into 12 equal "slices" representing each month of the year (Webb, 2010). Months with more deaths are shown with longer wedges so that the area of each wedge represents the number of deaths in that month from wounds, disease, or other causes. In the second year of the war, deaths from disease were captured in a similar graph, and proved deaths were significantly reduced, indicating the Sanitary Commission had improved hygiene in the camps and hospitals at the start of March 1855 (Webb, 2010).

CASE STUDY 2.2 (*continued*)

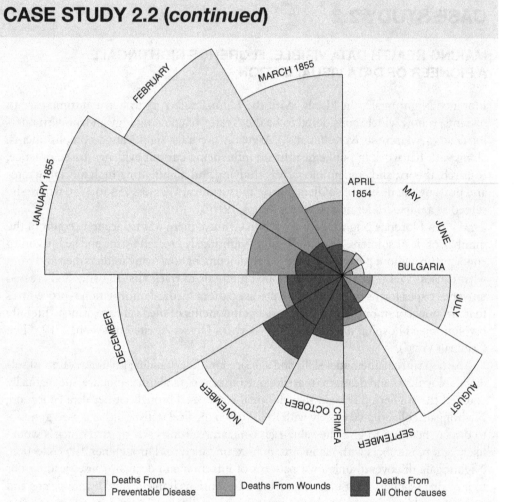

| Deaths From Preventable Disease | Deaths From Wounds | Deaths From All Other Causes |

Figure 2.6 The causes of mortality in the Army of Bulgaria and East Crimea 1954 to 1955—Baseline data.

Source: Adapted from Webb, C. (2010, June 3). *Florence Nightingale, data visualization pioneer.* Retrieved from http://www.stateoftheusa.org/content/florence-nightingale.php

This type of graphical statistical representation is common today, but in the 1800s it was revolutionary and marked Nightingale as a pioneer of data visualization (Lewi, 2006). Florence Nightingale showed the increase and differences in soldier mortality rates over a year within the diagram. While she was not the first to employ circular diagrams of this sort, she utilized it in a visually impactful way of showing her data. Nightingale used data to recreate the diagram and historians of statistics have found her visualization to be on point (Webb, 2010, "Famous for Data Visualizations"). Florence Nightingale's commitment and meticulous data analysis led to fundamental policy reforms after the war. Nightingale's skill in effectively utilizing the statistical method in army sanitary reform had led to her election, in 1858, to fellowship in the Royal Statistical Society, and in 1874, the American Statistical Association elected her an honorary member (Kopf, 1916).

Without understanding the essential characteristics of Big Data, how they are classified and sequenced for processing, and their quality, scientists and clinicians will find it difficult to utilize Big Data in the healthcare ecosystem. Visual representations of critical clinical outcomes, financial return on investment, and validation of models and processes of care are crucial to depict output and subsequent results of data analyses. Big Data storage, manipulation, and analysis, not without challenges, bring value to healthcare and nursing in the application of emerging technologies in practice and serve the Quadruple Aim.

NURSES AND BIG DATA

Nurses create **small data** every day in all care environments, including, but not limited to, EHRs, mobile health devices, digital sensors, radiology or nurse-driven assessment images, telehealth video, and ultrasound audio files. Collection of data occurs everywhere along the care continuum, including consumer-generated data (characteristics of Big Data are described in the "Data Characteristics" section). Produced in mass quantity, nurses collect these data as discrete facts described objectively without context or interpretation, and these healthcare data on their own have little value, as they are merely representations of the clinical environment, interventions, procedures, and items (Matney, Maddox, & Staggers, 2014). When data, such as a patient's fluid input and output and radiology results, are put into perspective and organized, information materializes; manipulation of this information results in a structured way (Matney et al., 2014). Nurses, perhaps unknowingly, create and use Big Data in all clinical and administrative environments, from the frontline staff to leadership at the middle and executive levels. Data in EHR discrete and indiscrete fields, such as clinical notes, as well as any remaining paper charting used for procedures, treatments, and health information management (HIM) purposes, along with enterprise resource planning systems (ERPs), are essential information for both patients and nurses and feed emerging technologies. While not aggregating them as would scientific data analysts, nurses process Big Data, taking the information generated from data and synthesizing it to create knowledge and guide interventions and decisions at the point of care and in administrative processes.

Opportunities

Big Data and data science have the potential to provide greater richness in understanding patient phenomena and in tailoring interventional strategies that are patient-centered (Brennan & Bakken, 2015), and to encourage personalized care, patient engagement, and innovation in care delivery and administrative processes. To advance the vision of a transformed health system, we need enhanced coordination in which quick and safely shared information happens among patients, consumers, clinicians, and interprofessional care teams to enable improved outcomes, quality of care, and lower costs. This vision requires access to real-time, accurate, and actionable health information (Sensmeier, 2015). Nursing at large needs to maximize the benefits of Big Data to advance the vision of promoting human health and well-being. However, current practicing nurses and nurse scientists often lack the required skills and competencies necessary for the essential use of Big Data (Topaz & Pruinelli, 2017). We strive for data-informed nursing practice, in which clinicians caring for patients have a greater understanding of the patient experience through data science. This desire imparts a more comprehensive view of the patient to devise creative approaches to interventions and monitor their outcomes (Brennan & Bakken, 2015). Nursing's participation in the Big Data and data science initiatives now underway is imperative to ensure that the discoveries from data not only shape our profession's unique understanding of the patient experience but also that the findings lead to knowledge that nurses find useful (Brennan & Bakken, 2015). The field of data science should inform all practicing nurses. It is the glide path to the future through partnerships and team science (Brennan & Bakken, 2015). There is an opportunity to transition nurses into data scientist roles to manipulate data sources to uncover patterns and bring action-able data-driven insights to life (Brennan & Bakken, 2015), as well as develop visualizations to show the value of Big Data. To accomplish that, nurses working with Big Data will need to draw from other disciplines, such as human–computer interaction and graphic design, to be able to develop appropriate visualization methods (Topaz & Pruinelli, 2017) that show the value of nursing, and outcomes attributed to nurses and providers in the current value-based care environment.

Adoption and Application of Data-Driven Emerging Technologies

Understanding Big Data characteristics, classification, processing, and visualizations is imperative. However, a solid comprehension of how data feeds emerging technologies such as The Internet of Things, Artificial Intelligence, Predictive Analytics, Virtual and Augmented Reality, Genomics, and Blockchain is also necessary and will lead to adoption and application of these technologies now and in the future. By embracing and applying these Big Data emerging technologies, nurses add value to nursing practice and the profession by harnessing innovation, what products, models, and processes are needed now that will create what's next in nursing, such as medical devices, novel workflows, and the transformation of whole health systems. Emerging technologies have already been introduced to the nursing practice ecosystem and all stakeholders and practicing clinicians are reaping the benefits of machine-driven, predictive, semantic, immersive, connected, and person-centered emerging technologies such as those discussed in this text.

Among multiple healthcare organizations, nurses represent the largest technology user group (Cassano, 2014). With more knowledge about how emerging technologies operate, nurses will be the purveyors of adoption and application of novel technologies, the influencers for all clinicians and administrators to do the same, and optimize nursing practice and administrative processes now and move into the next phases of care innovation. With that, nurses increasingly need to be experts at information management to stay current, including using emerging technologies and advanced analytics to show value in the healthcare ecosystem. In an industry where knowledge doubles every 12 months (Corish, 2018), nurses can no longer be the keepers of knowledge. Instead, they must become the masters of collecting and sharing that knowledge with others (Huston, 2013). Nursing education during the 20th century is no longer adequate for dealing with the realities of healthcare in the 21st century (Institute of Medicine, 2011). As patient needs and care environments have become more complex, nurses need to attain requisite competencies to deliver high-quality care, including leadership, health policy, system improvement, research and evidence-based practice, and teamwork and collaboration (Huston, 2013). Evolving to this, the new reality will occur through the steadfast adoption and application of emerging technologies with nurses at the forefront of life-changing innovations for both patients and nurses.

CONCLUSION

Evaluation of the extent to which nurses successfully serve the Quadruple Aim—including managing populations, impacting care outcomes, demonstrating a financial return on investments in value-based care—to improve both the patient and the nurse experience is scarce, but imperative to discover. Nursing practice drives value, and nurses have a direct and intimate influence on the quality, safety, and costs of patient-centered care (Pappas, 2013). Utilizing Big Data allows nurses to foster the fundamental shift brought on by Big Data thinking and the relevance that the answer to data questions must occur at the point of use rather than at the point of collection. What is important is not just the data, but the insights and scientific discoveries enabled by it (Brennan & Bakken, 2015). Nurses are already beginning to apply Big Data-enabled innovative technologies in practice and operations and noticing a positive impact on new value-based care programs, models, and approaches to show nurse value in the transforming healthcare environment to serve the Quadruple Aim. The chapters ahead will deal with the current state, exposure, and highlights of how Big Data feed emerging technologies on the leading edge today and how they are used to optimize patient care delivery.

GLOSSARY

Big Data: Data sets whose size is beyond the ability of typical database software tools to capture, store, manage, and analyze.

Nurse Value Drivers: Operational factors in value creation, with assets being both tangible and intangible and including intellectual and economic capital, nursing knowledge, revenue, efficiencies, and patient care outcomes, to align objectives, harmonize professional goals, guide industry investment, and identify financial worth.

Quadruple Aim: A framework developed to improve health through managing patient populations, reducing costs, improving patient satisfaction and engagement, and enhancing the well-being of practicing clinicians.

Small Data: Produced in mass quantity, nurses collect these data as discrete facts described objectively without context or interpretation, and these healthcare data on their own have little value, as they are merely representations of the clinical environment, interventions, procedures, and items.

Social Determinants of Health: Conditions where people live, learn, work, and play concerning a wide range of health risks and outcomes.

Value-Based Care: Cost over quality, with the "value" in value-based healthcare stemming from measuring health outcomes against the cost of delivering outcomes.

Vs of Big Data: The elements of enormity, function, diversity, performance, and usability of large data sets.

THOUGHT-PROVOKING QUESTIONS

1. How do the new value-based programs, models, and approaches directly influence daily tasks in your care setting?

2. Understanding the 10 Vs of Big Data, in what ways do these characteristics make you think differently about how you feed the data-rich healthcare ecosystem? Provide a detailed response.

3. What types of data visualizations are currently developed and utilized in your care environments?

4. In your clinical or nonclinical professional setting, understanding the Big Data life cycle, to what extent do you envision nurse's involvement in the adoption and application of emerging technologies?

REFERENCES

Aiken, L. H., Cimiotti, J. P., Sloane, D. M., Smith, H. L., Flynn, L., & Neff, D. F. (2011). Effects of nurse staffing and nurse education on patient deaths in hospitals with different nurse work environments. *Medical Care, 49*(12), 1047–1053. doi:10.1097/MLR.0b013e3182330b6e

American Nurses Association. (2015). *Nursing informatics: Scope and standards of practice.* Silver Spring, MD: Author.

Arthofer, K., & Girardi, D. (2017). Data quality-and master data management—A hospital case. *Studies in Health Technology and Informatics, 236,* 259–266. doi:10.3233/978-1-61499-759-7-259

BHM Marketing. (2016, October 11). *Value-based payment models and the future of healthcare—BHM Healthcare Solutions.* Retrieved from https://bhmpc.com/2016/10/value-based-payment-models

Brant, J. M. (2015). Bridging the research-to-practice gap: The role of the nurse scientist. *Seminars in Oncology Nursing, 31*(4), 298–305. doi:10.1016/j.soncn.2015.08.006

Brenan, M. (2018). *Nurses again outpace other professions for honesty, ethics.* Retrieved from https://news.gallup.com/poll/245597/nurses-again-outpace-professions-honesty-ethics.aspx

Brennan, P., & Bakken, S. (2015). Nursing needs Big Data and Big Data needs nursing. *Journal of Nursing Scholarship, 47*(5), 477–484. doi:10.1111/jnu.12159

Bresnick, J. (2017, June 5). *Understanding the many V's of healthcare Big Data analytics.* Retrieved from https://healthitanalytics.com/news/understanding-the-many-vs-of-healthcare-big-data-analytics

Carroll, W., & Hofmeister, N. (2018). *Predictive analytics and the impact on nursing care delivery* [Slide Show File]. Retrieved from http://365.himss.org/sites/himss365/files/365/handouts/550229529/handout-NI2.pdf

Caspers, B., & Pickard, B. (2013). Value-based resource management: A model for best value nursing care. *Nursing Administration Quarterly, 37*(2), 95–104. doi:10.1097/NAQ.0b013e3182869e17

Cassano, C. (2014). The right balance—Technology and patient care. *Online Journal of Nursing Informatics, 18*(3). Retrieved from https://www.himss.org/right-balance-technology-and-patient-care

Centers for Medicaid and Medicare Services. (2018). *Value based programs.* Retrieved from https://www.cms.gov/Medicare/Quality-Initiatives-Patient-Assessment-Instruments/Value-Based-Programs/Value-Based-Programs.html

Cianelli, R., Clipper, B., Freeman, R., Goldstein, J., & Wyatt, T. (2016). *The innovation road map: A guide for nurse leaders*. Retrieved from https://www.nursingworld.org/globalassets/ana/innovations-roadmap-english.pdf

Corish, B. (2018, April 23). Medical knowledge doubles every few months; how can clinicians keep up? *Elsevier*. Retrieved from https://www.elsevier.com/connect/medical-knowledge-doubles-every-few-months-how-can-clinicians-keep-up

Covell, C., & Sidani, S. (2013). Nursing intellectual capital theory: Implications for research and practice. *The Online Journal of Issues in Nursing*, *18*(2). Retrieved from http://ojin.nursingworld.org/mainmenucategories/anamarketplace/anaperiodicals/ojin/tableofcontents/vol-18-2013/no2-may-2013/nursing-intellectual-capital-theory.html

Cox, M., & Ellsworth, D. (1997, October 18–24). *Application-controlled demand paging for out-of-core visualization. Proceedings of the 8th Conference on Visualization '97, Phoenix, AZ*. Retrieved from https://www.nas.nasa.gov/assets/pdf/techreports/1997/nas-97-010.pdf

Delaney, C. W., Weaver, C. A., Warren, J. J., Clancy, T. R., & Simpson, R. L. (2017). *Big Data-enabled nursing: Education, research and practice* (pp. 118–119). Cham, Switzerland: Springer Nature.

Dhar, V. (2013). Data science and prediction. *Communications of the ACM*, *56*, 64–73. doi:10.1145/2500499

Donovan, F. (2019, May 8). *Organizations see 878% health data growth rate since 2016*. Retrieved from https://hitinfrastructure.com/news/organizations-see-878-health-data-growth-rate-since-2016

Feder, S. L. (2018). Data quality in electronic health records research: Quality domains and assessment methods. *Western Journal of Nursing Research*, *40*(5), 753–766. doi:10.1177/0193945916689084

Finkler, S. A. (2008). Measuring and accounting for the intensity of nursing care: Is it worthwhile? *Policy, Politics, & Nursing Practice*, *9*(2), 112–117. doi:10.1177/1527154408319452

Firican, G. (2017, February 18). *The 10 Vs of Big Data*. Retrieved from https://tdwi.org/Articles/2017/02/08/10-Vs-of-Big-Data.aspx?Page=2

Gintautas, D., Kurasova, O., & Žilinskas, J. (2013). *Multidimensional data visualization: Methods and applications*. New York, NY: Springer.

Gotz, D., & Borland, D. (2016). Data-driven healthcare: Challenges and opportunities for interactive visualization. *IEEE Computer Graphics and Applications*, *36*(3), 90–96. doi:10.1109/MCG.2016.59

Grimes, S. (2013, August). *Big Data: Avoid 'Wanna V' confusion*. Retrieved from https://www.informationweek.com/big-data/big-data-analytics/big-data-avoid-wanna-v-confusion/d/d-id/1111077

Healthcare Information and Management Systems Society. (2017, March 15). *Unlocking the data needed to drive population health efforts*. Retrieved from https://www.himss.org/news/unlocking-data-needed-drive-population-health-efforts

Huesch, M., & Mosher, T. (2017, May 4). *Using it or losing it? The case for data scientists inside health care*. Retrieved from https://catalyst.nejm.org/case-data-scientists-inside-health-care

Huston, C. (2013, May 31). The impact of emerging technology on nursing care: Warp speed ahead. *The Online Journal of Issues in Nursing*, *18*(2). Retrieved from http://ojin.nursingworld.org/MainMenuCategories/ANAMarketplace/ANAPeriodicals/OJIN/TableofContents/Vol-18-2013/No2-May-2013/Impact-of-Emerging-Technology.html

Institute of Medicine. (2011). *The future of nursing: Leading change, advancing health* (pp. 85–162). Washington, DC: National Academies Press.

Kopf, E. (1916). Florence Nightingale as statistician. *Publications of the American Statistical Association*, *15*(116), 388–404. doi:10.2307/2965763

Lewi, P. (2006). Florence Nightingale and the polar area diagrams. *Speaking of Graphics.* Retrieved from http://www.datascope.be/sog/SOG-Chapter5.pdf

Manyika, M., Chui, M., Brown, B., Bughin, J., Dobbs, R., Roxburgh, C., & Byers, A. H. (2011). *Big Data: The next frontier for innovation, competition, and productivity.* Retrieved from https://www.mckinsey.com/business-functions/digital-mckinsey/our-insights/big-data-the-next-frontier-for-innovation

Matney, S., Maddox, L., & Staggers, N. (2014). Nurses as knowledge workers: Is there evidence of knowledge in patient handoffs? *Western Journal of Nursing Research, 36*(2), 171–190. doi:10.1177/0193945913497111

McGonigle, D., & Mastrian, K. (2017). *Nursing informatics and the foundation of knowledge* (4th ed., p. 85). Burlington, MA: Jones & Bartlett.

Miller, H. D. (2009). From volume to value: Better ways to pay for health care. *Health Affairs, 28*(5), 1418–1428. doi:10.1377/hlthaff.28.5.1418

Mohanty, H., Bhuyan, P., & Chenthati, D. (2015). *Big Data: A primer* (p. 4). New Delhi, India: Springer.

Monsen, K. A., Peterson, J. J., Mathiason, M. A., Kim, E., Lee, S., Chi, C.-L., & Pieczkiewicz, D. S. (2015). Data visualization techniques to showcase nursing care quality. *CIN— Computers Informatics Nursing, 33*(10), 417–426. doi:10.1097/CIN.0000000000000190

New England Journal of Medicine—Catalyst. (2017, January 1). *What is value-based healthcare?* Retrieved from https://catalyst.nejm.org/what-is-value-based-healthcare/

Nurse Theory. (2018). *Nurse entrepreneur.* Retrieved from https://www.nursetheory.com/nurse-entrepreneur

Nursing Knowledge: Big Data Science Conference. (2018). *2018–2019 National Action Plan.* Paper presented at 2018 Conference Proceedings, Minneapolis, MN. Retrieved from https://www.nursing.umn.edu/sites/nursing.umn.edu/files/2018_proceedings.pdf

Office of the National Coordinator for Health Information Technology. (2008). *Promoting interoperability.* Retrieved from https://www.healthit.gov/topic/meaningful-use-and-macra/meaningful-use-and-macra

Pappas, S. (2013). Value, a nursing outcome. *Nursing Administration Quarterly, 37*(2), 122–128. doi:10.1097/NAQ.0b013e3182869dd9

Pappas, S., Davidson, N., Woodard, J., Davis, J., & Welton, J. (2015). Risk-adjusted staffing to improve patient value. *Nursing Economic$, 33,* 73–79.

Pappas, S., & Welton, J. (2015). Nursing: Essential to healthcare value. *Nurse Leader, 13*(3), 26–29. doi:10.1016/j.mnl.2015.03.005

Planning Tank. (n.d.-a). *Data processing—Meaning, definition, steps, types and methods.* Retrieved from https://planningtank.com/computer-applications/data-processing

Planning Tank. (n.d.-b). *Data processing cycle—With stages, diagram and flowchart.* Retrieved from https://planningtank.com/tag/data-processing-cycle

Rutherford, M. (2008). The how, what, and why of valuation and nursing. *Nursing Economic$, 26*(6), 347–351, 383.

Rutherford, M. (2010). The valuation of nursing begins with identifying value drivers. *Journal of Nursing Administration, 40*(3), 115–120. doi:10.1097/NNA.0b013e3181d04297

Salmond, S., & Forrester, D. A. (2016). Nurses leading change: The time is now! In D. A. Forrester (Ed.), *Nursing's greatest leaders: A history of activism.* (pp. 269–286). New York, NY: Springer Publishing Company.

Salmond, S., & Echevarria, M. (2017). Healthcare transformation and changing roles for nursing. *Orthopedic Nursing, 36*(1), 12–25. doi:10.1097/NOR.0000000000000308

Sensmeier, J. (2015). Big Data and the future of nursing knowledge. *Nursing Management, 46*(4), 22–27; quiz 27–28. doi:10.1097/01.NUMA.0000462365.53035.7d

Shafer, T. (2017, April). *The 42 V's of Big Data and data science.* Retrieved from https://www.elderresearch.com/blog/42-v-of-big-data

Smith, M., Saunders, R., Stuckhardt, L., & McGinnis, J. M. (Eds.). (2013). *Best care at lower cost: The path to continuously learning health care in America*. Washington, DC: National Academies Press.

Topaz, M., & Pruinelli, L. (2017). Big Data and nursing: Implications for the future. *Studies in Health Technology and Informatics, 232*, 165–171. doi:10.3233/978-1-61499-738-2-165

University of Minnesota School of Nursing. (2019). *Welcome to Big Data: Empowering health*. Retrieved from http://www.nursingbigdata.org/Home

U.S. Department of Health and Human Services: Health Resources and Services Administration. (2014). *The future of the nursing workforce: National- and state-level projections, 2012–2025*. Retrieved from https://bhw.hrsa.gov/sites/default/files/bhw/nchwa/projections/nursingprojections.pdf

Webb, C. (2010, June 3). *Florence Nightingale, data visualization pioneer*. Retrieved from http://www.stateoftheusa.org/content/florence-nightingale.php

Welton, J. (2010). Value-based nursing care. *The Journal of Nursing Administration, 40*(10), 399–401. doi:10.1097/NNA.0b013e3181f2e9f4

Welton, J. (2015). Hospital nursing workforce costs, wages, occupational mix, and resource utilization. *The Journal of Nursing Administration, 45*(10, Suppl.), S10–S15. doi:10.1097/NNA.0000000000000247

Welton, J., & Harper, E. (2015). Nursing care value-based financial models. *Nursing Economic$, 33*(1), 14–19, 25.

Welton, J., & Harper, E. (2016). *Big Data and nursing care: "What would Florence say?"*. Retrieved from https://ana.confex.com/ana/ndnqi16/recordingredirect.cgi/oid/Handout1349/ANA%20Big%20Data%20Welton_Harper_Final_23Dec15.pdf

Westra, B., Clancy, T., Sensmeier, J., Warren, J., Weaver, C., & Delaney, C. (2015). Nursing knowledge: Big Data science-implications for nurse leaders. *Nursing Administration Quarterly, 39*(4), 304–310. doi:10.1097/NAQ.0000000000000130

Zaugg, J., Marchese, M., & Keller, B. (n.d.). Florence Nightingale, a pioneer in data management. *InVivo Magazine*. Retrieved from http://www.invivomagazine.com/en/focus/interview/article/81/florence-nightingale-a-pioneer-in-data-management

3

Artificial Intelligence

WHENDE M. CARROLL

CHAPTER OBJECTIVES

- Define Artificial Intelligence (AI) and its domains.
- Understand the value of clinical decision-making using predictive data.
- Explain the different types of systems that learn through experience.
- Identify specific considerations involved in data used in AI programs and outcomes.

CONTENTS

INTRODUCTION

Artificial Intelligence (AI) has a long history in many industries, revolution-izing the way humans, the end users of the technology, communicate, transact financially and socially, and retrieve information. With many definitions and a long history, one industry that stands to profit most from AI's ability to think humanly is healthcare, by disrupting the way all clinicians care for patients and by making care delivery and administrative decisions in all settings, in both clinical and nonclinical roles. As the market for AI blossoms, one profession, nursing, stands to reap its benefits by enabling safety and care quality by augmenting clinical decision-making to provide value in new models of care, as well as sup-port organized, critical thinking and the nursing process to ultimately serve the Quadruple Aim. This chapter will discuss various AI programs, including expert systems, predictive analytics, machines that learn through experience, and natural language processing (NLP). These domains of AI, when adopted and applied judiciously in practice, enable nurses and interprofessional care teams in healthcare organizations to take critical actions through quick and more precise retrieval of information to improve decision-making, as well as efficiencies to evolve care delivery.

DEFINITION OF AI

Nurses must go beyond knowing the basics about AI and how it surrounds us every day to understand at a foundational level what it is. The classic example of AI, perhaps the most widely discussed and understandable example, is robotics. Robotics is the science and technology behind the design, manufacturing, and application of robots, programmable mechanical devices that can perform tasks and interact with their environment, without the aid of human interaction (VEX Robotics, n.d.). But robotics, commonly used in healthcare, is only a single ap-plication domain of AI.

Multiple definitions of AI exist and, depending on the perspective, purpose, and need for its applications, AI serves different purposes and comes in various forms. In 1956, John McCarthy, known as the "father of computer science," coined the original term for AI as "the science and engineering of making intelligent machines" (Torres, 2016, para. 3). Building on that definition, a predominant, concise description of what AI can do is the aptitude exhibited by smart machines broken down into perceiving, thinking, planning, learning, and the ability to manipulate objects (Kumar, Shukla, Sharan, & Mahindru, 2018). Another description is also "the art of creating machines that perform functions that require intelligence when performed by people" (Kurzweil, 1990, p. 14). And yet an alternate definition, "[The automation of] activities that we associate with human thinking, activities such as decision-making, problem-solving, learning" (Bellman, 1978, p. 3), adds the human element to the study of smart machines. These last two definitions sum up what Russell and Norvig (2010, p. 2) state is the realm of "thinking humanly," that is, the reliability of human performance versus ideal performance, in which a machine does the correct thing given what it understands. Discussion of AI, for this text and its applications, applied that focus on thinking and acting humanly as they pertain most to what we desire from AI and what it can do in medicine; that is, automating and computing more as humans do for the disruption of care mechanisms for improved patient-centered outcomes and financial management for patients and healthcare organizations.

In modern discussions about AI and what it does today, we get our information on the smart technology literature in the form of short articles, blogs, online curriculum, tweets, and other social media content which serve to demystify AI by experts in information technology (IT), business, policy, and economics providing their own definitions. Startling headlines warn of machines being programmed to take over the world and decrease human resources through smart automation. In fact, what we've witnessed since the dawn of modern computing beginning in the 1980s (Press, 2016) is the rise of AI used in e-commerce, search engine and social media platforms, smart communications, and financial transactions, technology that is commonplace and useful in our daily lives to be more effective in human judgment and efficient with our time. In truth, we've embraced AI and created more jobs, advanced cleaner energy, enhanced food sourcing, and improved education at all levels, to name a few applications. Improvements in industries abound due to AI, and this includes healthcare.

HISTORY OF AI

The first studies and roots of AI began in the 17th century when cybernetics, the science of communication and control theory that is concerned especially with the comparative study of automatic control systems (such as the nervous system and brain and mechanical-electrical communication systems; Merriam-Webster, n.d.), became of interest to scientists theorizing the connection between man, machine, and logic (Newell, 1982). Newell posited that the fields of biology, psychology, philosophy, linguistics, neuroscience, mathematics, and engineering dominated specific phases in AI's history where the studies and discoveries led to modern AI (1982). At various periods, more modern developments and definitions in AI were solidified, specifically 1940 and forward when machine pattern recognition, algorithms, semantics understanding, robotics and tasks, and learning emerged. The desire for AI advancements accelerated quickly with the rise of science fiction literature, fueling the imagination of achieving human-like thinking with AI, and the introduction of personal computers in 1980 that made data storage and applications a reality for the growth of technology (Buchanan, 2006; Case Study 3.1).

The modern-day phase of AI focuses on machines that move and think smarter and can automate, to help humans make decisions and solve problems (Newell, 1982). One significant area scientists focus on to meet these industry imperatives is **expert systems**. The technique uses advanced computer programs that imitate the knowledge and reasoning capabilities of an expert in a particular discipline to develop a tool that a layman can use to solve difficult or vague problems. These systems contrast conventional computer programs as they combine

CASE STUDY 3.1

AI'S HISTORY: ALAN TURING AND A GAME OF CHESS

Two well-known studies challenging the legitimacy and fortitude of AI in the last century that aimed to test if machines can indeed think more intelligently and humanly have had mixed results. The first is the Turing Test, a central, terminal goal for AI research to conclude if humans will ever be able to build a computer that can sufficiently imitate a human to the point where a suspicious judge cannot tell the difference between a human and a machine (C. Smith, McGuire, Huang, & Yang, 2006). The second is the study of the ability for a machine to beat a human player at a chess game. Alan Turing, deemed "the father of modern computer science" (Hodges, 2014), a 20th mid-century mathematician in 1950, posed the question: Can machines think? (Turing, 1950). This inquiry was the precursor to modern AI as defined later by John McCarthy, whose further AI research focused on the basis that all aspects of learning or features of intelligence can explain the creation of a machine that mimics them (Torres, 2016). The advent of **deep learning** (DL) led to great strides in AI where computers could perform tasks that were deemed almost impossible previously, such as diagnosing certain diseases better than humans, and generating art in the style of grand masters. In 2019, the Turing Prize, sometimes called the "Nobel Prize of computing", was won by AI pioneers Yann LeCun, Geoffrey Hinton, and Yoshua Bengio (Piper, 2019). Pursuing the chess AI hypothesis has been worthy, and one that has been "solved" by AI researchers by producing programs that can outplay the world's best chess players. Still, the best game-playing machines did not understand the concepts of the game and merely relied on brute force approaches to play (C. Smith et al., 2006). The advent of DL changed all that, where a DL system considers only a small set of moves, just like a human grandmaster, while playing chess, and is still able to beat the best human players (Silver et al., 2018).

facts with rules that assert relations between the facts to achieve a rudimentary form of reasoning equivalent to AI (World Information, n.d.). The three main facets of expert systems are (a) an interface that allows interaction between the system and the user, (b) a database or knowledge base that consists of rules, and (c) the inference engine, a computer program that executes the computational process. These systems bridge past theoretical AI research with modern practice; however, their shortcomings include the management of unforeseen events, in application, as they must describe every encountered condition. Also, they are limited to narrow problem domains such as medical image interpretation, but still have the advantage of being more cost-effective than paying an expert or a team of specialists (World Information, n.d.).

As can be seen in the history of research and development of AI, challenges abound, even while advances are being made rapidly in many industries, including healthcare. The fantasy of intelligent machines still lives as we accumulate evidence of the complexity of intelligence (Buchanan, 2006). Through the years,

John McCarthy's optimism and commitment to the fact that machines can and will, in the future, think remained strong. He posited that the "speed and memory capacity of today's computers may be insufficient to stimulate many of the more complex functions of the human brain" and that the main obstacle is not the lack of a machine's competency, but the "inability to write programs that take full advantage of what we have" (McCarthy as cited in Torres, 2016, "A Legend"). With AI, this is where science remains today with the need for human resources and knowledge that will further the advanced analytics innovations including those that accurately predict future events and process unstructured human language.

History of AI in Healthcare

Inklings of the usefulness of AI in medicine began in the early 1970s when researchers began to develop computer programs for clinical decision-making. During that time, a small group of medical computing research groups concurrently realized that the field of AI offered potential solutions to problems that had previously constrained the effectiveness and acceptance of formerly researched medical decision-making programs of the 1960s (Gorry, 1984). Upon reviewing the systems developed in the prior decades, Gorry (1984) encompassed a primary concern with the construction of AI programs that performed diagnosis and made therapy recommendations. Unlike medical applications based on other programming methods, such as purely statistical and probabilistic methods, the basis of medical AI domains will begin to use symbolic models of disease entities and their relationship to patient factors and clinical manifestations (Gorry, 1984). The impetus of cumulative AIM (AI in medicine) programs stemmed from the fact that a clinician confronted with a potentially ill patient did not have sufficient information then to decide on a diagnosis or therapeutic management. He or she did, however, have general medical knowledge and experience, enabling a formulation of some speculative hypotheses about the state of the patient's health (Gorry, 1984). This opinion exerted a considerable effect on the strategy the clinician employed in dealing with the patient, but provided options to the physician such as tests and treatments (Gorry, 1984). This strategy was the dawn of the clinical decision support (CDS) systems that exist today (Kulikowski, 2015).

Since that time, other domains of AI have gained steam in robotics, image recognition, and implementation of electronic health record (EHR) systems for clinical support and improved workflow. The first documented robot-assisted surgical procedure, a percutaneous brain computed tomography-guided biopsy, was performed in 1985 (Marino, Shabat, Gulotta, & Komorowski, 2018), although automation in robotics surgery is yet to be employed and they remain mostly manipulated by humans. Research is ongoing on how the next robot generation will store and utilize Big Data from patients and procedures to reproduce steps using its self-learning ability, similar to solutions already used in the park-assist technology in automobiles (Marino et al., 2018). Like robotic surgery, the rise of image recognition for radiology has also come to the forefront as an everyday use of AI in image processing and interpretation using **machine learning** (ML; Pesapane, Codari, & Sardanelli, 2018), which will be discussed later in this chapter.

Vyborny and Giger began researching uses of AI in mammography in 1994, stating "the well-trained radiologist brings far too much insight and versatility to the diagnostic process … to be casually relegated to a secondary role" (Vyborny & Giger, 1994). Today, while computed tomography and magnetic resonance imaging are the top modalities of AI's focus, these are followed closely by digital x-ray, mammography, fundus imaging of the eye, ultrasound, and echocardiography (S. Shah & Joffe, 2018). Late stage EHRs are beginning to leverage AI algorithms, to convert rules-based CDS systems with limited data sources to machine-driven solutions, and to fundamentally improve data discovery and extraction and personalize treatment suggestions, with the potential to make EHRs more user friendly (Davenport, Hongsermeier, & Alba McCord, 2018). A critical goal is to simplify hard-to-use EHRs, which are frequently cited as contributing to clinician burnout (Downing, Bates, & Longhurst, 2018). Today, customizing EHRs for a clinician's ease of use is mostly a manual process, and the system's rigidity is an obstacle to care process improvement. AI, and ML specifically, will help EHRs continuously adapt to users' preferences, improving both clinical outcomes and clinician well-being ((Davenport et al., 2018).

AI'S PROMISE IN HEALTHCARE

The use of AI in healthcare, as is already being witnessed, will go far toward turning data into useful and actionable information that benefits the health and care of patients (Sensmeier, 2017), and transforming the workforce through augmenting administrative processes in healthcare organizations. AI has substantial implications for the healthcare industry, perhaps more so than others (Stanford Medicine, 2018), as the McKinsey Global Institute estimates that 15% to 20% of the healthcare market has the potential to be impacted by AI, making it one of the most affected sectors (Batra, Queirolo, & Santhanam, 2018). AI healthcare spending is expected to reach $6.6 billion by 2021, with an annual growth rate of 40% between 2014 and 2021; meaning the health AI market in medicine will have grown more than 10 times (Frost & Sullivan, 2016). Intelligent computing has the potential to add a significant amount of value by improving care quality, specifically by allowing for quicker and more precise diagnoses, higher quality treatment plans, and new ways of managing processes (Stanford Medicine, 2018).

Some of the most anticipated advances in AI that equate to net positive benefits include prediction of diagnoses and risk profiling, such as for chronic and acute disease, readmissions, and adverse events. Also, identifying care variation leads to more effective care planning and pathways for patients, personalizing care by optimizing best practice, such as clinical pathways; increasing patient access to care; reducing cost; improving outcomes for patients; and enhancing the well-being of clinicians (Stanford Medicine, 2018), particularly nurses. In addition to reducing human error, AI will aid in personalizing treatments through mining genomics claims, social media, sensor, and wearable technology data; gaining clinical knowledge; improving efficiencies; and enhancing CDS inside and outside of EHRs (Sensmeier, 2017). With these applications, we can utilize AI to lower costs, decrease waste and unnecessary care, and decrease variability and lack of standardization, while improving healthcare organization infrastructure in our value-based care environment, increasing efficiencies and productivity, and decreasing silos.

With the judicious use of AI, and what it can do as a driver of value and innovative transformation to advance the future of healthcare, the technology holds great promise to enhance several aspects of the care process, including personalizing treatments to maximize effectiveness, monitoring population health and outcomes, and discovering new evidence that will inform care delivery. Nurses' charge is to integrate the human aspects of care while automating reasoning processes (Sensmeier, 2017) as we seek to comprehend, adopt, and utilize AI in nursing care settings.

What AI Is

At first glance, foundational concepts of AI can appear overwhelming and noisy. In modern literature and urban descriptions of AI, many scientists and writers, in a rush to explain the concepts and uses of AI, move quickly to describe it as ML. While ML is an application of AI that is the basis of data processing for AI (to be discussed in the chapter), in truth there are many functions of AI (see Figure 3.1). Expert systems and robotics (discussed previously in this chapter) in NLP, vision and speech analytics, and those designed specifically for planning, scheduling, and optimization also exist today, among many others that are emerging.

What falls under the umbrella of AI is the basis of the technology nurses use every day, personally and in all care environments with digitalized smart devices such as cell phones, web search engines, multiple social media and e-commerce platforms, various kitchen appliances, messaging systems, and chatbots. In programming AI there is a straightforward process that requires minor complexity to automate machines. To begin to uncomplicate and understand AI programming,

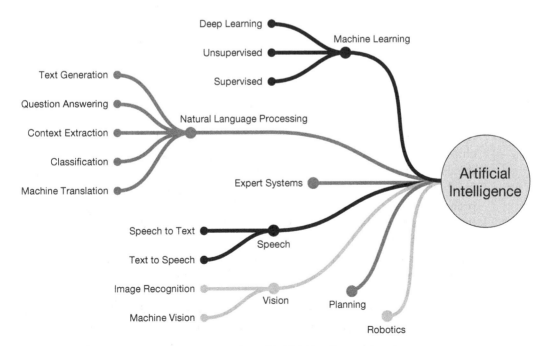

Figure 3.1 An overview of Artificial Intelligence domains.

nurses can begin to understand that algorithms are at the technology's core. **Algorithms** are sequential instructions that ensure particular task completion. They are a set of well-constructed rules given to an AI program to help it self-learn when it encounters a trigger, that is, an event or behavior resulting from the instructions of the intermeshed algorithms. When several algorithms are put together and layered in applications, they become the backbone of AI (Polson & Scott, 2018). The subsequent layering of algorithm groups results in many algorithms that can transform and create new algorithms in response to learned inputs and data as opposed to relying only on the inputs it was designed to recognize as triggers—this ability to change, adapt, and grow based on new data is known as "intelligence" (Ismail, 2018).

In healthcare, AI becomes "clinical intelligence," machine algorithms designed for medical diagnostic and treatment processes utilized in the appropriate use cases for patients, everyone in a healthcare organization, and payers; it is an extension of care for the right treatment, to the right person, at the right time. This use of AI in the clinical space leads ultimately to "precision intelligence," smart machines that work better for everyone along the care continuum (Healthcare Information and Management Systems Society [HIMSS], 2018). Nurses' use of AI enhances care delivery and administrative processes that decrease healthcare costs through better operational efficiencies and billing, improve the revenue cycle and supply chain management, enable a focus on quality outcomes by managing populations of people through risk stratification of cohorts with chronic diseases, and lower lengths of hospital stays and hospital readmissions. AI in action also enhances the patient experience, heightening engagement and satisfaction and improving the nurse experience through balancing patient loads, impacting distracting human factors while providing care, and increasing human interaction through optimizing the EHR, allowing for more time with people, thus serving the Quadruple Aim. In short, AI in healthcare is machine algorithms, through learning, perceiving, planning, and more in-depth understanding of language processing, which are used to suggest recommendations for clinical decision-making that is smarter, faster, and more precise.

What AI Is Not

AI algorithms and the machine are not standalone and built solely from wires, chips, nuts, and bolts. Programming of AI applications is not possible without the data at their core to help them learn, evolve, and grow. One of the holdups in adopting AI is that the amount of information needed to process and comprehend it is so unsustainable that it is difficult to expect the average clinician to integrate the bulk of it into his or her daily decision-making efficiently, with accuracy (Bresnick, 2017). For effective clinical decision-making, Big Data must feed programs for algorithms building from many healthcare sources, including the EHR; medical claims; voice, audio, and imaging files; and workforce and care setting throughput data such as enterprise resource planning to include bed management and human resources. The fundamental and intrinsic/structural and critical characteristics of the data and the successful use of them in AI is essential to succeeding at building smart machines as they must be as complete, structured, cleaned, and unbiased as possible (Carroll, 2019a). With that, more data are best as the number of robust datasets help machines to learn, predict, and process semantic languages better. Building on small datasets is possible, but more AI programs work more successfully with voluminous data (Ng, 2019).

Smart machine outputs should not automatically "do" for humans; they should be adjunct supportive tools that act as assistants to enhance judgment. The products of AI applications are no longer simple search engines relaying results in computer programs, which was one of the early functions of AI programs, such as web search engines (Polson & Scott, 2018). AI mechanisms are evolving into new smart suggestion and recommendation machines that drive decision-making. While clinical and precision intelligence mechanisms largely are now machine-driven and better automate processes for specific applications, it is important to note that it is also "assistive intelligence"; utilization of AI should augment or supplement care instead of replacing the humans who provide it. The transforming technology outputs suggestions requiring human judgment to apply AI recommendations to be helpful and strike a balance with data-manipulated science and decision-making (HIMSS, 2018). The output of AI should not default actionable decision-making. Their design should provide the most appropriate care and make the best decisions through its move to smart suggestions and recommendations, with human judgment at its side, "rather than act like death robots that are controlling the entire healthcare ecosystem" (McGrane, 2018); this is why machine automation will not eliminate jobs, including nursing roles, as some suggest (Manyika et al., 2017). AI's advantage is that it can work 24/7 without breaks, vacations, or complaints; however, algorithms are not programmed to be empathetic, and will not replace the significant judgment and use the critical thinking only elicited and given by humans to provide the most appropriate patient care (Topol, 2019). Smart machines won't wholly replace laborers but will instead reallocate resources and duties that ultimately impact how nurses work, transform essential roles, decrease low-value tasks, and allow time for high-value interactions and work that is useful for nurses' unique clinical and operational skills and abilities.

AI CONSIDERATIONS

With the advancement of AI in clinical decision-making for diagnosing disease, using collaborative robotics for procedures, and redefining clinical and administrative processes, nurses must take a deliberate approach to view the effects of technology on patients and society. These include careful consideration of policy, health equity, bias (as discussed in Chapter 1, Emerging Technologies and Healthcare Innovation), data privacy, governance, and security with the techniques used for algorithm building and their applications. According to the Executive Office of the President, National Science and Technology Council Committee on Technology in 2016, AI's presence and advancement in society are driven by "three mutually reinforcing factors: the availability of big data … dramatically improved machine learning approaches and algorithms … and the capabilities of more powerful computers" (Skiba, 2017, p. 108). With this, a study completed by The MITRE Corporation looking at the implications of

AI in healthcare recommended that the technology should address a significant, identified clinical need, and must perform at least as well as the existing standard approach. Further, substantial clinical testing needs to verify the performance of the new technology under the wide range of clinical situations, and AI should provide improvements in patient outcomes, patient quality of life, and practicality in use (The MITRE Corporation, 2017). These suggestions are imperative with companies in a "rush to market" approach developing and marketing AI solutions, to first evaluate the actual return on investment and the real clinical value they bring to patients and populations. Both assessment and regulation are essential to protect patients and ensure access and fairness with the technology.

Policy and Ethics

Two national agencies and associations have drafted policies to recognize the exceptional opportunity to ensure that the evolution of AI in healthcare benefits patients and the community. In the United States, S.2806—National Security Commission on Artificial Intelligence Act of 2018, introduced to the Senate in May 2018—directs legislatures to form a commission to consider the methods and means necessary to advance the development of AI. These include ML and associated technologies to comprehensively address the national and economic security needs of the country, including economic risk, and any other related issues (Congress.gov, 2018), including healthcare needs. Likewise, policy drafted by the American Medical Association (AMA) in 2018 aims to advance the ethical and technical specifications of AI to promote the development of thoughtfully designed, high-quality, clinically validated healthcare. The association posits the design and evaluation of AI should consider best practices in user-centered design, particularly for all members of the healthcare teams; is transparent; and conforms to leading standards for reproducibility. Moreover, the policy encourages AI developers to take a design approach that identifies and serves to address bias, avoids introducing or exacerbating healthcare disparities including when testing or deploying new AI tools on vulnerable populations, protects all individuals' privacy interests, and preserves the security and integrity of personal health information (AMA, 2018).

Bias and Equity

The opportunity for bias exists in building AI algorithms for healthcare communities and how they are used, developed, implemented, and applied for the most appropriate medical care (discussed in Chapter 1, Emerging Technologies and Healthcare Innovation). In AI, development bias can be vetted out early on, but only if a diverse group of people critically consider the problem from conceptualizing a project (Gershgorn, 2018) and the outcomes. With the transition into this time of clinical intelligence, AI developers, clinicians, and patients must be prudent about subjectivity and inclusivity in the data being used to make life-altering healthcare decisions (Stanford Medicine, 2019). In healthcare, biased outcomes mean one group of people get better medical treatment than another based on characteristics of gender or race, but sometimes because of other traits, like language, skin type, genealogy, or lifestyle (Gershgorn, 2018). This is especially true with the potential of age and gender bias, an example being in clinical trials where many psychological and social science studies are composed of participants who are Western and educated, and from industrialized, prosperous, democratic countries where men, over women, are favored as participants; the highest population, approximately 67%, are college students (Stanford Medicine, 2019).

Further, studies also routinely leave out female and elderly populations, as well as those with additional conditions that require medical interventions, such as pregnant women; these individuals are often excluded entirely (Hart, 2017). This disparity is especially true in less-connected rural communities where poorer and older members of society don't have access to the digital technologies that can be used to improve healthcare, such as AI, and are not included in the subsequent health and social data. Looking to the future when accessibility to treatments and technological tools will be available, it may be too late, as the AI algorithm programming will have used younger, more urban bodies (Hart, 2017).

Datasets that contain patient-specific data are only as good as those populations that we extract data from for AI algorithm building. And lacking the rich socioeconomics data, such as the Social Determinants of Health, make inequity and bias more prevalent. Critically looking at ethics and data objectivity in AI cannot be deferred to a future activity as AI developers have begun to use their technologies for providing both second opinions and alternative options in medical practices (Gershgorn, 2018). Recognizing and mitigating bias in AI systems is essential to building trust between humans and machines that learn, and as AI systems find, understand, and point out human contradictions, they also unearth where we are partial, narrow-minded, and cognitively biased, leading us to adopt more fair or equal views of smart machines. In the process of recognizing our bias and teaching machines about our shared values, we may improve not only AI, but also ourselves (IBM Research, n.d.).

Regulation and Governance

The United States and other developed countries use different strategies to ensure the regulation of AI programs and the data protection and security that govern them. Some feel that particular global jurisdictions, most notably the United States, believe in a more "soft-touch, self-regulatory" approach than the European Union (EU; Chen et al., 2018). In the United States, AI falls under medical device regulation by the U.S. Food and Drug Administration (FDA). As of 2019, control is limited to medical device safety and development aiming to use judicious yet expedited approaches to move AI solutions to market. During 2018 many intelligent technologies were approved by the FDA (Mulero, 2019; see Table 3.1) for clinical use, including applying image recognition for early detection of diabetic retinopathy and wrist fractures (FDA, 2019b).

The FDA has made strides to pre-classify novel technologies for appropriate use and safety for patients (FDA, 2019a), as well as establish a Pre-Certification (PreCert) pilot program for establishing processes for software as a medical device (SaMD), which may include software functions that use AI and ML algorithms,

Table 3.1 FDA Approved and Cleared AI-Powered Devices, 2017 to 2018

Company	Approval Date	Indication
Arterys	January 2017	MRI heart interpretation
Alivecor	November 2017	Atrial fibrillation detection via smart watch
MaxQ-AI	January 2018	CT brain bleed diagnosis
Arterys	February 2018	Liver and lung cancer (MRI, CT) diagnosis
Viz.ai	February 2018	CT stroke diagnosis
Imagen	March 2018	X-ray wrist fracture diagnosis
Icometrix	April 2018	MRI brain interpretation
IDx	April 2018	Diabetic retinopathy diagnosis
Neural Analytics	May 2018	Device for paramedic stroke diagnosis
Bay Labs	June 2018	Echocardiogram ejection fraction determination
Zebra Medical	July 2018	Coronary calcium scoring
iCAD	August 2018	Breast density determination (mammogram)
Aidoc	August 2018	CT brain bleed diagnosis
Apple	September 2018	Atrial fibrillation detection

Source: Reproduced with permission from Topol, E. J. (2019). High-performance medicine: The convergence of human and artificial intelligence. Nature Medicine, 25, 44–56.

within FDA's current authorities (Mulero, 2019). However, in contrast to other countries, FDA mandates for citizens' AI-related data security and privacy, as well as software regulation, to protect personal health data and information; AI automation on subjects remains in development (Rowe, 2019).

In contrast, the EU has drafted comprehensive legislation to protect its citizens' data adequately and to emphasize the use and consequences of intelligence automation by implementing the General Data Protection Regulation (GDPR). The mandate seeks to create full transparency rights, and safeguards against automated decision-making, a fact that EU leaders believe AI developers who manage the data of intelligent solutions and users must understand. One Article of the GDPR grants individuals the right to contest a completely automated decision if it has legal or other significant personal effects, with the regulation also requiring technology companies to inform customers about the general functionality of an automated system when decisions are made using those data (Chen et al., 2018). The GDPR also acts as a safeguard to personal healthcare data and information, folding in additional mandates, such as those of the United States Health Insurance Portability and Accountability Act of 1996 (HIPAA). These include managing and ensuring the integrity and security of large amounts of data, demonstrating compliance with the requirements involving controllers and processors, and overseeing the compliance efforts of suppliers (Jensen, 2018).

AI AND NURSING

AI is a novel concept in healthcare, particularly in nursing practice. However, AI is gaining traction in the profession, and nurses, as the largest population of healthcare workers, are the primary end users in intelligent technologies. AI and nursing are leading enhancements in standardizing patient care processes and workflows to improve quality of care, impact cost, and optimize the patient and provider experience. The success of once revolutionary technologies such as EHRs, mobile health, telehealth, and remote patient monitoring sensors and education simulation has been proven. Their ability to deliver high-quality, safe patient care, which is now conventional technology used in care delivery and education, along with new data-driven, intelligent innovations in the healthcare space will further clinical capabilities and add value to patients, nursing, and healthcare at large. Nurses, in tandem with divergent collaborations between healthcare organizations with big and small technology companies—startups, incubators, and spin-outs—growing the healthcare AI space (discussed in Chapter 1, Emerging Technologies and Healthcare Innovation), now infuse Big Data-enabled solutions for more reliable disease prediction, amplified semantic language comprehension, and voice recognition (Carroll, 2019a).

The time is now to transform practice using intelligent and emerging technologies as healthcare solutions for new models of care, processes, and products to continue to advance practice and successfully further care quality and safety initiatives. As the Institute of Medicine (IOM) stated in its landmark paper in 2010, "[h]ealth care organizations should engage nurses and other front-line staff to work with developers and manufacturers in the design, development, purchase, implementation, and evaluation of medical and health devices and health information technology products" (Institute of Medicine, 2010, p. 11). This imperative will bring forth the understanding of the voices of the patient, the nurse, clinicians, and healthcare administrators by including nurses early in the process of the design and development of these types of innovations, not only as the "end users" but also as the knowledge bearers of the intricacy of the patient care environment (Clipper, Batcheller, Thomaz, & Rozga, 2018). As valued members of design, adoption, and implementation teams, nurses working along with the technology experts have helpful insight that can leverage their knowledge of patient care and administrative needs and recognize the best use cases for AI to meet the goals that clinical intelligence can bring to the care environment. Nurses have expertise and skill sets that are unique and can influence the development and adoption of these technologies and prevent costly mistakes that arise from lack of healthcare user input (Clipper et al., 2018). Along with learning about emerging technologies and partnering with data science teams, nurses should engage in leadership roles for technology innovation to encourage the commencement of AI. Nurse leaders will foster and manage the changing roles that support novel technologies as end users, nurse scientists, and developers, and in other areas of healthcare where nursing's valuable knowledge is needed, as their roles emerge and evolve with the onslaught of AI.

A fundamental contribution that nurses can make to the progress of AI in healthcare is in providing standardized data. Patient care and administrative data include comprehensive elements of patient assessment, care planning, intervention, and outcomes. Once standardized to provide complete, clean data, these will improve knowledge about care management along the care continuum for a compilation into the processing of large datasets in AI programs. These standardized data are a viable driver of AI development in healthcare as it is an opportunity not only for nurses but also for patients to be represented in this evolution (Risling, 2018). Nurses' collection of structured data for the development of clinical intelligence stimulates knowledge creation, management, and a move toward understanding and wisdom. When data are discrete, clean, and complete, it can add context in an AI program. The knowledge derived from data and connected information from nurses helps machines to begin to learn, perceive, and plan and subsequently start to understand and apply wisdom for utilization as smart suggestions for real-world clinical decision-making, in many cases becoming faster, more accurate, and more precise. With more data, the process continues, and machines become smarter and help nurses better use human judgment to provide the most appropriate decision-making and care processes.

AI and Support of Patient-Centeredness and Safety in Nursing Practice

Despite the introduction of AI at a rapid pace in healthcare, its effect on desired practice and significant benefits in all care settings is still limited and will need further research. As mentioned, the adoption and implementation of now successful daily utilization of once revolutionary healthcare technology give promise to the present and future success of AI and nursing. Comprehension of the foundations of AI, the symbiotic nature of it along with how it supports and enhances nursing practice, is essential with its increased use in practice in today's value-based care environment. Embracing AI will prove advantageous, with nurses having it at their fingertips for better clinical decision-making, as it will improve nurses' value in health systems as providers and payers look to health IT innovations, including AI, to disrupt the business model of healthcare and the products and solutions offered to meet the Quadruple Aim (see Chapter 2, Nursing Value and Big Data; Carroll, 2019a).

As noted, AI programs have moved from merely searching for results to smart suggestion and recommendation machines (Polson & Scott, 2018), and for nurses' benefit, they now guide decision-making by enhancing critical thinking and the nursing process, which enables pattern detection and semantics understanding and processing that ultimately thinks more like humans in clinical environments. The fruits of AI are tools that provide for better clinical practice and administrative processes, including enhanced computerized alerts and reminders, clinical guidelines, condition-specific order sets, focused patient data reports and summaries, documentation templates, diagnostic support, and contextually applicable clinical reference information (McLean, 2018). In nursing practice, the end goal of emerging technologies such as assistive intelligence is to decrease the low-value tasks that can be automated by smart machines to allow more high-value activities and best use of nurses' essential skill to give more time with patients to improve their experience engagement and satisfaction. As nurses seek to improve serving patient needs, there is a strong belief that AI can be critical in this ongoing care evolution through saving time and resources to optimize patient care delivery. AI has the potential to disrupt how care is delivered on many fronts, saving time on unnecessary activities and indeed providing nurses more time with patients for other care needs (EchoNous, 2018).

In all clinical care environments, the opportunities for errors, adverse events, and near misses are endless. With all clinicians and specific to nursing are the human factors that lead to unsafe practice environments, and AI can aid the vulnerabilities and strengths of human performance. Threats to safe nursing practice include nurses experiencing high patient loads (Aiken et al., 2011), alarm fatigue, too much technology, unfamiliarity with the task at hand, inadequate time, poor communication, underestimation of risk, poorly designed workflows, and reliance on memory (Tocco, 2013). Intelligently designed algorithmic workflows that make patients and nurses safer in instances where the clinical environment or potential interventions may be harmful should be made available. Safety can be maximized through enhanced AI CDS system tools to decrease the chances of drug–drug interactions, duplicative treatments, and care variation; identify risks for hospital-acquired infections and conditions; and determine the most appropriate staffing levels to improve safety in a care setting and patient outcomes. One path to using these tools effectively for safe, quality care is the advancement of safety algorithms and complementary use of AI with critical thinking and the nursing process. With this, the understanding of how AI and its use can impact and enhance nurses' decision-making by supporting critical thinking and positively impacting the nursing process is imperative.

AI, Critical Thinking, and the Nursing Process

AI impacts human factors and organized thinking in the practice environment; nurse's critical thinking and the nursing process do as well, each complemented by the recommendations and suggestions of smart machines. Overall the multifaceted and complex elements of critical thinking applied in nursing practice create a nonlinear exercise that focuses nurses on clinical decision-making (Paul & Heaslip, 1995). It helps meet the broad criteria for evaluation of the clinical process when delivering care, those being the standards of care nurses strive for by national nursing associations and entities such as the American Nurses Association Scopes and Standards of Practice and The Joint Commission patient safety goals and core measures. Critical thinking is a flexible, fluid process, guiding nurses to learn to think and to anticipate what will happen next and concluding which interventions to apply with each patient, by asking the critical what, why, and how questions (Carroll, 2019b) in practice. Also, AI supports information synthesis, the reasoning process by which nurses reflect on and analyze personal thoughts, actions, and decisions, as well as those of others (Paul & Heaslip, 1995). AI used in tandem with critical thinking strengthens nurses to generate new knowledge, look beyond the obvious of what is happening with the patient, and challenge traditional ways of thinking used in practice historically (Paul & Heaslip, 1995). The fluid process of reasoning is enhanced by AI; the use of smart machines is balanced with nurses' unique skill sets and solid clinical knowledge, using human judgment throughout the process (Carroll, 2019a).

The nursing process works in parallel with critical thinking. It is a systematic, phased approach that is used by nurses to gather data points, critically examine and analyze those data, evaluate patient response, develop a plan for action, take the appropriate action, then evaluate the effectiveness of interventions and measure subsequent outcomes (Johansen & O'Brien, 2016). AI, together with critical thinking and human judgment, significantly impacts all phases of the nursing process by increasing the speed and accuracy of evaluation, anticipation, and knowledge synthesis generation (Carroll, 2019a). The assessment phase of the nursing process is the vital collection and verification of data that are analyzed and communicated to members of the healthcare team and patients (Johansen & O'Brien, 2016). AI helps this step through the processing of data inputs and intelligent extraction of patient-specific data to more accurately determine the patient's condition. Diagnosis, defining the patient disease state that allows a nurse to individualize care, and planning, the stage where nurses customize care priorities and determine interventions, are two of the steps where AI programs also expedite nursing practice. Next, the intervention phase, when the actions necessary for achieving the goals and outcomes to assure they get initiated and completed occurs (Johansen & O'Brien, 2016), is where AI gets put into motion using data from multiple patient and healthcare data sources to inform actionable recommendations specific to each patient. Finally, AI strengthens evaluation to help nurses refine priorities and collect data on an ongoing basis (Johansen & O'Brien, 2016). Throughout these phases, the data inputs processed by smart machines help nurses reiterate the full process by accelerating the initiation of findings, plans, actions, and outcomes; enabling the patient-centered practice; and suggesting the best clinical decisions throughout the care continuum (Carroll, 2019a).

PREDICTIVE ANALYTICS

Understanding that multiple sources of healthcare data are rapidly feeding the ocean of Big Data and the precious need for the volume of those data to develop AI algorithms will help move to the next phase in the drive to realize a value-based change in nursing. As the largest group creating clinical data, nurses have the most significant opportunity to standardize them at the point of care to ensure the structure of data that feed the ecosystem primes the environment for AI algorithm building. EHRs, medical devices, and sensor technology that collect data into discrete fields are the catalyst for realizing clinical and precision intelligence. As technology matures and we begin using AI, nurses should be able to obtain information only once and see it reused often (Cipriano & Hamer, 2013). This premise evolves nursing care to where we are now, proving the ability to use data to uncover rich patterns within them through technical automation to drive change in nursing care delivery and administrative processes. It is instrumental in fostering a culture of inquiry among the workforce, giving frontline nurses access to data to enable a scholarly approach to change and transformation that emphasizes research and evidence-based practices (Anderson & Patterson, 2013) to serve the Quadruple Aim ultimately. Used judiciously, nurses can count on emerging technologies, such as smart machines that use prediction to push the latest best practices and research-based evidence to the point of care, enabling them to make even the most complex clinical decisions with a high degree of confidence (Simpson, 2012), accuracy, and efficiency.

Predictive analytics falls under the umbrella of AI. It is a mathematic approach that uses statistical computations to analyze historical data from multiple sources to predict future events. This advanced analytics methodology refines those data, using the information to extract hidden value from newly discovered patterns that dynamically inform data-driven decision-making to proactively know what will happen, when it will happen, and what to do about it (Bari, Chaouchi, & Jung, 2017). In healthcare, predictive analytics through ML and DL is now used to predict who will get sick, when, and how nurses will treat patients. Further, prediction in healthcare supports organizational processes for making administrative decisions that impact nursing care (Sensmeier, 2017). The goal is to intervene in decision-making earlier (now) rather than later (when it's too late), such as with diagnosing sepsis, identifying chronic disease progression—such as diabetes—and determining the best nurse staffing levels to add essential value to patient care delivery.

Predictive Analytics' Purpose

The well-constructed rules that are the foundation for machine algorithms used in predictive analytics are not unlike the standard rules used by nurses in formal and informal clinical decision-making. The difference is the addition of layering algorithms into the smart machines now used in clinical settings. Before AI, methods for forecasting patient diagnosis and treatment in nursing included using more simplistic CDS tools such as the Modified Early Warning System (MEWS) to help recognize patient deterioration (Carroll, 2019b). Advanced analytics transform these types of CDS tools in that they become more intelligent in precision decision-making at the unit level and the bedside. Beyond using these rules-based pre-intelligent tools, layered algorithms now hyper-drive CDS tools in medical devices and EHRs currently used in practice. They enhance the accuracy and speed at which nurses can take action in determining patient deterioration and hospital throughput bottlenecks. as well as the best care planning and discharge approach to ensure seamless transitional care to decrease hospital readmissions and high clinic and emergency department utilization, which improve patient experience and quality and reduce healthcare costs (Bates, Saria, Ohno-Machado, Shah, & Escobar, 2014).

In complex healthcare environments, nurses make clinical decisions every day with the help of critical thinking, intuition, and following the nursing process (Carroll, 2019a). Despite this, with lack of tactical ability to bring together the health Big Data sources available in a care setting, nurses may still guess or use heuristics, described as "mental shortcuts commonly used in decision making that can lead to faulty reasoning or conclusions" (Elstein, 1999 as cited in Marewski & Gigerenzer, 2012, p. 81). Heuristics are in large part used due to the inability to synthesize data in the hectic environments and an overreliance on limited information, pattern recognition, experience, and initial impressions (Klein, 2005). Clinical decisions based on heuristics alone overlook correct diagnoses, appropriate intervention, and outcomes. Hindsight is a common type of heuristics attribute, an overestimation of the probability of a diagnosis or event after obtaining knowledge of the correct diagnosis or event, where manual case review may help with mitigating future occurrences and decisions (Klein, 2005). Leveraging advanced analytics such as predictive algorithms, or models, with human clinical heuristics adds potency—speed, reliability, and organization—in clinical decision-making.

The Value of Predictive Data and Analysis

Four types of data used for analytics exist in the spectrum of healthcare— descriptive, diagnostic, predictive, and prescriptive, which advance from simple to more complex (Gartner, 2016; see Figure 3.2). Based on this, for nurses, the use of these types of data in decision-making increases in value moving from descriptive to prescriptive data. Descriptive data tell us what happened and diagnostic data tell us why something happened. Both provide past tense information or hindsight. In our clinical settings, nurses readily see this information in clinical reports and dashboards that require data analysts and clinicians to query systems to discover causes for past events. Hindsight uncovers missed opportunities for care or process improvements. Moving to the use of predictive data helps nurses pre-emptively discern what events will happen, why, and when they will happen. The strategy of using data in this way provides insight, by better understanding anticipation of what interventions are needed to ensure an event does or does not occur to make decisions proactively. Predictive data used in CDS systems designed to mitigate patient deterioration, and errors, adverse events, or near

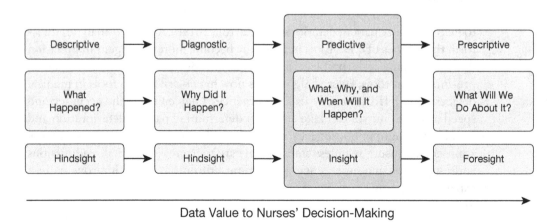

Data Value to Nurses' Decision-Making

Figure 3.2 Data types, purpose, and value in decision-making.

Source: Gartner. (2016). *2017 planning guide for data and analytics.* Retrieved from https://www.gartner.com/binaries/content/assets/events/keywords/catalyst/catus8/2017_planning_guide_for_data_analytics.pdf

misses, demonstrate this in practice. Layered with intelligent algorithms, predictive data advance to the use of prescriptive data, which allow nurses to ensure more precisely what to do about events beforehand to administer the most appropriate, evidence-based practices and standards for better outcomes. The subsequent foresight that prescriptive data impart empowers nurses to move beyond hindsight and provides insight to use information, knowledge, and wisdom along the path of data complexity. The advancement along the spectrum from simple to more intricate data enables enhanced data analysis from less to more difficult to promote randomized testing, predictive modeling through intelligent algorithm use, and forecasting to optimize care and processes (HIMSS, 2019).

DECISION-MAKING USING PREDICTIVE DATA: INPATIENT LENGTH OF STAY

To highlight the value of using basic to complex data to identify the best interventions that lead to quality outcomes, consider the example of using prediction for the appropriate patient length of stay (LOS) in the inpatient setting upon patient admission. When a patient enters the hospital, if nurses use descriptive and diagnostic data alone to determine LOS, it will likely be an uninformed decision, forcing heuristics to merely guess how long a patient may or should stay, based on perhaps only an admitting diagnosis code estimating what might be appropriate or reasonable. With the hindsight that this creates, looking backward is the sole method for nurses to analyze these data through reports and dashboards to show trends, including how long a patient stayed—for too long or not long enough. The sources and actions that led to the outcomes prompt the need to drill down in standard or ad hoc reports if the patient has a delayed discharge, or hospital readmission resulting from an early discharge.

In contrast, predictive analytics can determine inpatient LOS using automation and smart machine algorithms to determine the appropriate or reasonable LOS based on data-driven patterns from multiple Big Data sources that alert nurses of what to expect as the most beneficial time frame from the first contact with the patient. Nurses can then be prescriptive through the patient's hospital journey. With foresight, applying evidence-based interventions more quickly is possible, including discharging the patient if he or she has been in the hospital for too long, to decrease the risk of hospital-acquired conditions and increase patient satisfaction, and identifying if the patient is not staying long enough, to prevent a hospital readmission or emergency department visit. With insight and foresight, nurses can anticipate the best LOS to plan and take necessary actions earlier, allowing more time for precision treatments and therapies that can reduce them. Knowledge, gained through prediction, enhances nurses' ability to provide high-quality care planning coordination and determine breakdowns in hospital flow, such as long radiology wait times or poor bed management, and make adjustments as needed, including canceling a discharge or readjusting staffing to improve care for all hospital patients throughout the continuum of care.

Machine Learning

ML, a branch of AI (Iriondo, 2019), is the study of computer algorithms and programs said to improve automatically through experience concerning a class of tasks and performance measures (Mitchell, 1997). Specifically, with predictive analytics, ML is a set of algorithms (models) that can take a set of data inputs (variables and features) and return a prediction (Caffo, Leek, & Peng, 2016). ML differs from traditional statistical analysis for prediction, in that statisticians cast confidence more often on data modeling, and that ML methods focus more on the predictive models' accuracy (Breiman, 2001). This distinction is vital as nurses may wonder why statistics are not used in clinical and administrative settings for intelligent prediction. Statistics underscore inference, the process of using data analysis designed to deduce the characteristics or properties of a population; in contrast, ML smart machines automatically learn over time through experience, emphasize predictions, evaluate results via prediction performance, and serve to highlight algorithm performance and robustness of outcomes (Caffo et al., 2016). A simple analogy for ML is that it is the equivalent of teaching a system the rules of a game and getting the program to practice it at elementary and intermediate levels. After preparation and further training, the system can, in real time, play at advanced levels (Bari et al., 2017).

ML is well suited for using complex healthcare data, data in various forms collected from multiple sources, and data that are voluminous for prediction. While data mining, the process used to extract usable data from a broader set of any raw data (The Economic Times, n.d.), can unearth previously unknown connections in data, ML categorizes the new and upcoming unknowns, learns from them based on its previous processing of the data, and gets better at incorporating them into known data (see Figure 3.3). Both techniques lead to richer insight and improved understanding of the data (Bari et al., 2017). There are four techniques of ML, and each has its own approach based on the business problem that needs to be solved, as well as the amount, type, and volume of the data (Hurwitz & Kirsch, 2018).

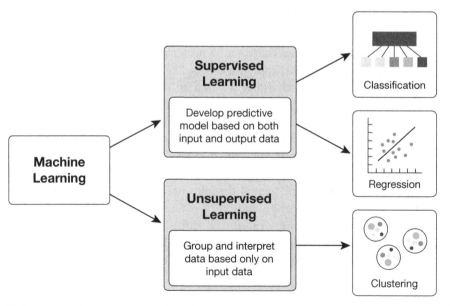

Figure 3.3 Two types of classic machine learning methods. Supervised learning, which trains a model on known input and output data to predict future outputs, and unsupervised learning, which discovers unknown patterns or basic structures in input data.

Source: MathWorks. (2019). *What is machine learning? How it works—Techniques & applications.* Retrieved from https://www.mathworks.com/discovery/machine-learning.html

SUPERVISED LEARNING

In **supervised learning**, machines build prediction models based on evidence in the presence of uncertainty from both input and output data (Figure 3.4). A supervised learning algorithm takes a known set of input data and known responses to the output data and trains a model to generate reasonable predictions for the answers to new data (MathWorks, 2019). This learning technique is used most commonly when known data for the output data have labels that define their meaning (Caffo et al., 2016). To develop predictive models, supervised learning uses classification and regression techniques. Classification models classify input data and discrete output for predictions, for example, whether a tumor is benign or cancerous. Typical applications include medical imaging and speech recognition, including voice clinical charting or dictation. Classification algorithms data can be tagged or divided into specific groups or classes. Regression approaches predict continuous responses, for example, changes in a patient's temperature or variations in blood pressure. Scientists use regression techniques when working with a numeric output variable or if the nature of the response is a real number, such as values from vital signs, lab results, or the precise time until failure for a piece of equipment (MathWorks, 2019).

UNSUPERVISED LEARNING

Unsupervised learning discovers hidden patterns or basic structures in data. It is used to draw inferences from datasets consisting of input data only, without labeled responses. This technique allows the computer to learn how to do something and use this to determine structure and patterns in data; for example, trying to uncover unobserved factors in unlabeled data, such as image recognition

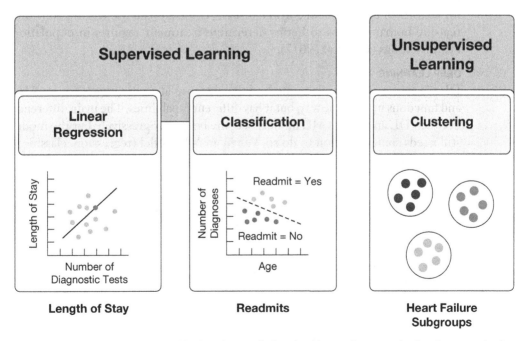

Figure 3.4 Outputs of common machine learning prediction algorithms using supervised and unsupervised learning for length of stay, readmits, and heart failure subtypes.

Source: Qureshi, I. (2018, October 26). *Healthcare data scientists: 6 steps for utilizing your data analysts.* Retrieved from https://www.healthcatalyst.com/insights/healthcare-data-scientists-steps-leveraging-data-analysts

processing, where recognition techniques are used for image data segmentation (Holehouse, n.d.). It is known as "unsupervised" because there is no standard or benchmark outcome to judge against for the prediction outputs, segmenting data into groups of features; this may be used before moving the predictive outputs to a supervised learning approach (Caffo et al., 2016). Clustering is the most common unsupervised learning technique (Figure 3.4). It is used for exploratory data analysis to find hidden patterns or groupings in data (MathWorks, 2019). Applications for cluster analysis include gene sequence analysis and scoring patient satisfaction results. Also, if an Internet of Things (IoT) health IT vendor wants to adjust the locations where he or she is placing sensors in a hospital unit for optimal connectivity and sensing, the vendor may use unsupervised ML to estimate the number of clusters of patients requiring the sensors for the best technical outcomes.

REINFORCEMENT LEARNING

Reinforcement learning (RL) is a type of behavioral model of ML technique that enables an agent, a piece of software in an AI program, to learn in an interactive environment through trial and error by using feedback from its own actions and experiences (Bhatt, 2018). Both supervised learning and RL use mappings between inputs and outputs. However, unlike supervised learning where feedback provided to the software program is a correct set of actions for performing a task, RL employs rewards and punishment as signals for positive and negative behavior (Alzantot, 2017). RL is different in terms of goals, compared to unsupervised learning. The goal in unsupervised learning is to relate data points; in RL, the purpose is to find a suitable action model that would maximize the total cumulative reward of the agent (see Figure 3.5; Bhatt, 2018). In clinical practice, for cohorts of patients with chronic disease, clinicians can use RL to determine real-life human actions to better determine treatment regimes in population health settings (Liu et al., 2017).

DEEP LEARNING

DL is a subset of ML and is a method that encapsulates cognitive learning, ML, and functions in the same way, but it has different capabilities. The main difference between DL and ML is ML models become better progressively but the model still needs some direction to do so. When an ML model (regression, classification, or clustering) returns an incorrect prediction, a scientist needs to fix that problem purposefully, but in the case of DL, the model will do it autonomously (Hariharan, 2018). DL is associated with an ML concept known as an artificial neural network (ANN), which is inspired from neurons in the human brain to

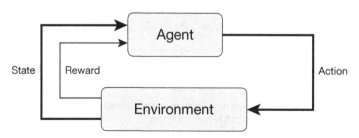

Figure 3.5 Process of reinforcement learning.

facilitate the modeling of arbitrary functions, requires a massive amount of data, and is highly flexible when it comes to modeling multiple outputs simultaneously (Jain, 2015). Neural networks (NNs), or nodes, were initially motivated by looking at machines that replicate the brain's functionality, with the hypothesis that the brain has a single learning algorithm and it can process and learn from data from any source (Holehouse, n.d.; see Figure 3.6).

Reasons for the increased popularity of DL today are the immense increase in chip processing abilities, the significantly increased volume of Big Data used for ML, and the recent advances in ML (Deng & Yu, 2014). This progress enables DL techniques to exploit complex datasets effectively, through nonlinear compositional functions, to learn distributed and hierarchical features that are domain-specific; these are used to describe the data and representations, a set of classifiers, or the language that a computer understands (Deng & Yu, 2014) to make effective use of both labeled and unlabeled data (Faggella, 2019). Research is now focusing on developing data-efficient ML, mainly DL systems that can learn more efficiently, with the same performance, quicker, and with fewer data. For cutting-edge nurse-led use cases that support precision healthcare, including chatbots, population health management, and genomics, abstraction helps to make sense of data such as images, sound, and text—an automatic car driving system is an example of DL (Deng & Yu, 2014).

The ML Process

The foundation of ML is to seek an answer to the question, "How can we build computer systems that automatically improve with experience, and what are the fundamental laws that govern all learning processes?" (Mitchell, 2006 as cited in Faggella, 2019, "How We Arrived at Our Definition"). The method of ML is a five-step process that involves obtaining input data, cleaning and preparing data, training data through the chosen algorithm(s), data testing and validating, and receiving and improving the output. Learning and improvement occur through the cyclic method of retraining and retesting data from ML outputs (Figure 3.7)

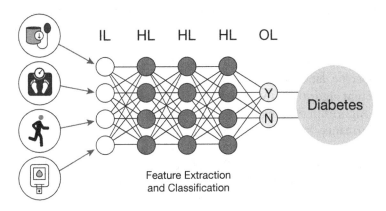

Figure 3.6 Deep learning artificial neural networks.

Cognitive intelligence algorithms process clinical data inputs (IN, input layer) through hidden layers of cells (HL) that adjust and connect based on well-constructed rules in a smart machine to perform a task, and subsequently develop responses (OL, output layer) based on pattern recognition similar to how a human's brain responds to external stimuli.

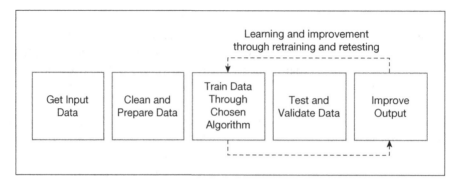

Figure 3.7 The machine learning process.

To begin the ML process, the initial, and arguably the most time-consuming, step is feature engineering, the process of collecting and manipulating datasets that will train the model. This step is critical because it determines the dataset labels, algorithmic logic, and ensures accurate connections during the cyclic process (Ng, 2019). Cleaning prepares data by removing irrelevant and redundant data; further, the methods of feature selection and extraction use only the most relevant data attributes and transform them into new formats that describe variants within the data and reduce the amount of information required to develop the ML model (Zhou, 2018). This stage is where, for example, extraneous and duplicative patient demographics, vital signs, and lab results from healthcare data pulled from multiple sources, such as from the EHR, medical claims, and data sensed through IoT devices, are scrubbed and fixed for dataset completeness.

Training the labeled dataset, once collected and prepared, entails choosing a model that best fits the use case. Commonly used algorithmic prediction models include linear and logistic regression, decision trees, random forest, gradient boosting, and neural networks (NNs), discussed later in this chapter. The size and dataset quality will determine each, as will the nature of the data, computational time availability, task urgency, and use case for the model (Le, 2019), and algorithm determination will generate various data visualizations. It is customary to trial several algorithms on a dataset to fine-tune them with slightly different parameters to identify variation in performance. Typically, most of the models perform similarly; however, the quality and underlying structure of the dataset for predicting the data outputs is essential, as an algorithm might perform well on specific datasets and poorly on others, which leads to the crucial need to trial different algorithms (Mastanduno, 2017).

Algorithm training will fit and tune data, and testing and validation of their performance is a key step toward precision learning and output improvement. Test datasets are separated as "unseen" data to evaluate the model. Data are always first split to determine reliability before training the model and are put aside until choosing the algorithm (Ng, 2019). Comparing test and training performance avoids overfitting when a model does not generalize well from training data to test data; this is the outcome if model performance is high on training dataset but poor on the test data, in which case it is overfit due to lack of original data structure and quality (Elite Data Science, n.d.). Improvements of unknown pattern recognition and outcomes including predictions materialize with rigorous dataset training and testing, after which machines begin to learn on their own.

DIFFERENCES BETWEEN ML AND DL

Like ML, DL completes feature extraction for processing and outputs, and the data are trained, tested, and validated. However, the DL technique uses an ANN architecture organized into layers composed of interconnected nodes. The nodes of the network perform a weighted sum of the input data that transfer to an activation function. Weights become dynamically optimized during the training phase (Pesapane et al., 2018). In DL, there are three different kinds of layers: the input layer, which receives input data, and the output layer, which produces the results of data processing, with hidden layer(s) in between. A deep ANN differs from the single hidden layer, NNs, or classical NNs, by having a large number of hidden layers, which characterize the depth of the network (Erickson, Korfiatis, Akkus, & Kline, 2017). DL avoids the design of a dedicated high-level feature extraction process from raw sensory data (Topol, 2019) by using a deep NN approach that automatically unearths and represents complex features as a compilation of simpler ones (Pesapane et al., 2018; Case Study 3.2).

CASE STUDY 3.2

PIECES TECHNOLOGIES

USING AI TO IMPROVE HOSPITAL PATIENT LENGTH OF STAY, READMISSIONS, AND DETERIORATION

Pieces Technologies, a health information technology (IT) spinoff of Dallas-based Parkland Center for Clinical Innovation, has developed an AI cloud-based software solution called DS (Decision Sciences) that uses language semantics processing and predictive modeling techniques to process both patients' clinical and social determinants data. The intelligent technology enables nurses to follow patients through their care journey and provide decision support across the care continuum (Cohen, 2018a), tackling high-risk social and clinical issues that can impact adverse outcomes, particularly during the hospital stay (Pieces Tech, 2018b).

Pieces DS is a cloud-based, back-end AI technology that predicts patients at risk for adverse outcomes and excess hospital utilization. The solution applies advanced analytics, using ML in conjunction with clinical human augmentation, as well as chart reviews by Pieces' clinicians, to ensure the highest accuracy in the predictive models. In addition to processing vast amounts of structured data, the DS language processing technology reads and interprets unstructured data such as free text progress and dictated notes for actionable insights. With this assistive intelligence, DS discovers critical patterns within the data, which enables the activation of precision, expedited interventions—the right care, the team member at the right time—for enhanced and efficient decision-making to maximize operational and clinical effectiveness, without overalerts improving human factors in practice (Pieces Tech, 2018b). DS continuously

(continued)

CASE STUDY 3.2 (*continued*)

monitors patient data for risk of readmission, overutilization of ED services, excessive LOS, and social determinants that may affect patient quality outcomes (Pieces Tech, 2018b). The platform's Clinician-in-the-Loop™ prediction and communication capabilities are evidence-based, clinically developed, and DS's configured ML algorithms that maintain, monitor, and continually improve in clinical practice, with demonstrated 80% to 95% positive predictive value (PPV), or precision; 80% to 95% sensitivity (true positive rate); and five times fewer false-positive results upon model testing and validation (Pieces Tech, 2018b).

PREDICTION FOR LENGTH OF STAY AND READMISSIONS

Despite efforts to prevent avoidable hospitalizations, research shows that 3.3 million patients are readmitted within 30 days of discharge, resulting in $17B of preventable costs annually (Pieces Tech, 2018b). Reducing readmissions and avoidable hospitalizations can have an immediate, positive impact on a hospital's bottom line. While multidisciplinary teams work to find solutions to this issue, many still lack actionable insights needed for precise results, particularly recognizing the importance of social determinants and their impact on avoidable readmissions. To improve outcomes, as an example, a major academic, integrated delivery network licensed a Pieces DS machine learning platform to sit atop their electronic health records (EHRs) and clinical data warehouses to predict and monitor the likelihood of costly clinical events including readmissions and excess LOS to identify at-risk patients. With the solution in place at several of their hospitals, the organization realized reductions in readmissions and LOS excess; the ability to discern where readmission efforts should be focused; more than 95% PPV identifying barriers to discharge, including pending tests, delayed provider consultant feedback, and unclear follow-up activities and post-discharge placement (Amarasingham, 2019); and more than 850 nursing review hours saved per year, per hospital (Pieces Tech, 2018b). Overall, the DS clinical decision support tools assist nurses in creating a holistic and personalized discharge plan, making smart recommendations in the patient's EHR (Miliard, 2018).

EARLY WARNING SYSTEMS FOR PATIENT DETERIORATION AND SEPSIS

With the use of Pieces intelligent technologies, The Parkland Center for Clinical Innovation, Pieces' nonprofit research affiliate, realizes the benefits of AI's ability to analyze massive volumes of data and alert clinicians up to 48 hours in advance of a patient requiring a rapid response team (RRT) for clinical deterioration (Miliard, 2018). While some hospitals use automated early warning systems (EWSs) from structured data and RRTs, these tools are often limited (Pieces Tech, 2018a). To improve response time and the opportunity window for care teams to intervene on patients at risk of deterioration, a study was conducted with a client hospital to evaluate the effectiveness of the machine learning, predictive solution. Researchers surveyed 4,600 encounters

(*continued*)

CASE STUDY 3.2 (*continued*)

in near real time with the Pieces Tech EWS prediction software to identify patients at risk of critical deterioration. The research found that the population mortality rate was 3.4%, and the ICU transfer rate was 3.9%. In this trial, the Pieces EWS intelligent technology identified an ICU transfer or death in one out of five cases. Further, 60% of the time if the patient died or transferred to the ICU, Pieces preidentified the individual, and among sepsis cases, approximately one out of two identified by Pieces Tech resulted in ICU transfer or death (Pieces Tech, 2018a).

This evidence shows that Pieces intelligent technology solution enhances nurse decision-making, improves patient outcomes by identifying hidden patterns in data including social determinants to optimize patient throughput, identifies risk of rehospitalization, monitors for critical conditions, and strengthens communication among care teams. This emerging technology improves the quality of nursing care delivery and safely and efficiently transitions patients into the community.

Natural Language Processing

Unstructured written and spoken communications generate one of the largest and critical sources of Big Data. For this reason, the emergence of a technical mechanism to capture those data and enable computers to understand better and process human (unstructured) languages, to move smart machines closer to a human-level understanding of semantics, is necessary and is already gaining prominence in the healthcare industry (Seif, 2019). **Natural language processing** (NLP), under the canopy of AI, is meeting this need. NLP is defined as the automatic manipulation of natural, unstructured language, like text and speech, through algorithmic programming (Gn, 2018). Combined with advanced analytics, NLP human–computer interaction enables scientists to develop algorithms for language translation, semantic understanding, and text summarization, making it easier to understand and perform computations on volumes of text with less effort (Seif, 2019). Examples of NLP are smart language translation software, automated question answering systems, and text correction applications (Kiser, 2016). In healthcare and nursing, applications include extracting EHR text from notes in non-discrete fields to use for CDS systems and patient clinical trial matching (Cohen, 2018b), and the extrapolation of text from scholarly literature to use as data sources for other healthcare AI programs (Carroll, 2019a).

NLP is a way for computers to analyze, understand, and derive meaning from human language in a relatively low-cost, efficient, and useful method and the basis for its algorithms is ML algorithms (A. Smith, 2018). Instead of hand-coding large sets of rules, NLP relies on advanced analytics, such as ML, to automatically learn these rules by analyzing a set of examples (i.e., a sizable text-based catalog, like a book, down to a collection of sentences), and making a suggestion or prediction. In general, the more data analyzed, the more accurate the model will be (Kiser, 2016). By utilizing NLP, developers can organize and structure knowledge to perform tasks such as automatic summarization, translation, named entity recognition, relationship extraction, sentiment analysis, speech recognition, and topic segmentation. Different from everyday word processor operations that treat text as a primary sequence of symbols, NLP deliberates the hierarchical structure of language—several words make a phrase, several phrases make a sentence, and, ultimately, sentences convey ideas (Kiser, 2016; see Figure 3.8).

To program and use NLP, the understanding of language is imperative. Text communication is different for various genres, including clinical notes, research papers, blogs, and social media platforms as they have different writing styles. Thus, there is a substantial component of surveying data manually to understand semantics, and how humans analyze them. When a human reasoning system, such as ignoring incorrect text in messages, using emojis to imply sentiment, and understanding the context of sarcasm develops in a machine, a consistent ML approach to automate that process and scale is possible (A. Smith, 2018). Scientists believe NLP is a domain in which DL will make a significant impact in the coming years. The expectations are that ANN systems will understand sentences or whole documents and improve when they learn strategies for selectively attending to one part at a time (LeCun, Bengio, & Hinton, 2015).

By harnessing NLP, AI can successfully mirror human speech, style naturally flowing sentences, and give human-to-machine interactions a personal touch (A. Smith, 2018). NLP is beginning to address two significant problems in healthcare—enabling better clinical documentation and providing insights from unstructured data in EHRs (Edwards, 2018). NLP's method of data mining integration in health IT systems allows nurses in all clinical settings to reduce subjectivity in decision-making and provide new, useful health-based knowledge. NLP programmed in conjunction with predictive algorithms supports best-in-class health knowledge and assists all clinicians to develop a set of precise and reliable forecasting for better informed decisions and improve the use of healthcare data

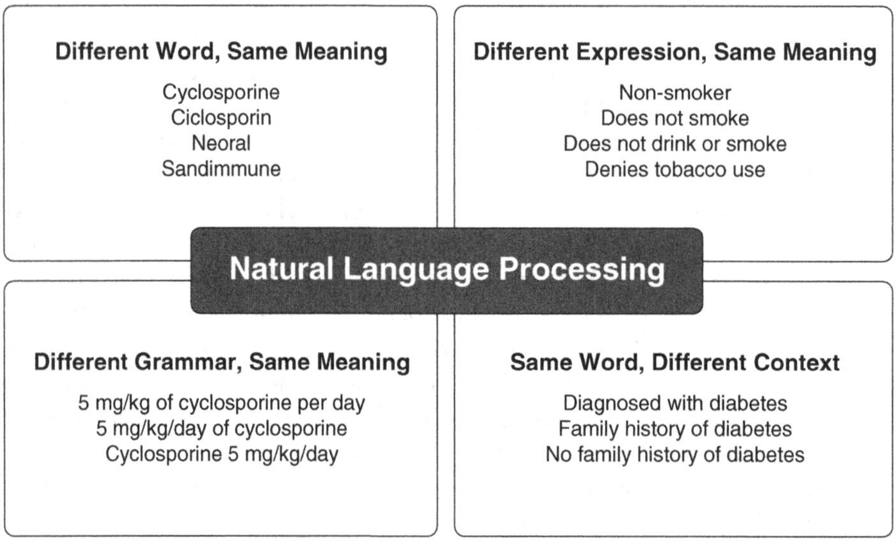

Different Word, Same Meaning

Cyclosporine
Ciclosporin
Neoral
Sandimmune

Different Expression, Same Meaning

Non-smoker
Does not smoke
Does not drink or smoke
Denies tobacco use

Natural Language Processing

Different Grammar, Same Meaning

5 mg/kg of cyclosporine per day
5 mg/kg/day of cyclosporine
Cyclosporine 5 mg/kg/day

Same Word, Different Context

Diagnosed with diabetes
Family history of diabetes
No family history of diabetes

Figure 3.8 Natural language processing can understand differences in grammar, expressions, and meaning to interpret sentence structures and reveal the underlying facts and relationships when used in clinical settings.

Source: Reed, J. (2016). *Gaining business insight for clinical trials—Text analytics for a data driven approach.* Retrieved from https://www.prismeforum.org/wp-content/uploads/2015/12/PRISME_Linguamatics_TextAnalytics_ClinicalData-Jane-Reed.pdf

along the nursing data value spectrum (descriptive, diagnostic, predictive, and prescriptive) for enhanced diagnosis and patient care (Bogdanov, 2019).

According to Cohen (2018b), there are several use cases of NLP in healthcare. These include speech recognition, clinical documentation improvement, data mining research, computer-assisted coding, automated registry reporting, clinical trial matching, CDS, risk adjustment, and hierarchical condition categories. And, in the future, using NLP for ambient virtual scribes, computational phenotyping and biomarker discovery, and population surveillance will become more prevalent (Cohen, 2018b). Health IT vendors, such as Pieces Tech in Dallas, Texas, are now developing nurse-specific NLP solutions that add beneficial CDS value propositions including those that assist with determining patient hospital LOS to ensure timely discharge and enhance transitional care to lower the incidence of hospital readmission (Pieces Tech, 2019). Nursing scientists have begun to study NLP related to processing of nursing and provider EHR clinical notes and diagnostic reports for identification of limb ischemia (Afzal et al., 2018), wound information (Topaz et al., 2015), mapping clinical terms for text extraction and reasoning (Zhou et al., 2011), Social Determinants of Health data (Gupta & Birch, 2019), medication reconciliation (Topaz & Pruinelli, 2017), and oncology treatments (Hyun, Johnson, & Bakken, 2009).

AI—A DEEPER UNDERSTANDING

AI algorithms can undoubtedly be more efficient, less expensive, and more accurate than humans. However, they can also be highly complex and opaque, and organizations that deploy AI may not fully understand the decisions that an algorithm arrives at (The Economist, 2018). In all industries there is a call to take pause and better comprehend algorithmic models interworking for the explanation of how they function, realize their actual performance, and identify how to interpret their outputs for rigor in practice, research, and education (Holzinger, Biemann, Pattichis, & Kell, 2017) not only in healthcare but for society at large (Ng, 2019). Although the trade-offs for the benefit of prediction in healthcare exist, experts posit that end users of AI and advanced analytics should not arbitrarily apply outputs and predictions without strong consideration (Topol, 2019).

Methods that generate data models can be difficult for scientists and end users to interpret as their functional form in relating the available input data to a given output is extremely complex in ML; in fact, AI algorithms are often characterized as "Black Boxes" (Vellido, 2019). Due to incomplete datasets, bias that can lie within them, other challenging facets of preparing data and algorithm training, and determining outputs, testing performance of an algorithmic model, particularly in healthcare where predictions potentially treat a large population outputs, requires thorough testing for quality, safety, and ethics (Topol, 2019). To fully trust outputs, it is first imperative to test model performance before applying results for true statistical function and probability determined by sensitivity, specificity, PPV, negative predictive value (NPV), and other measures of accuracy (Baratloo, Hosseini, Negida, & Ashal, 2015; van Stralen et al., 2009).

Predictions and recommendations made by AI-based systems can be wrong, or not right enough (Lipton, 2016), for instance, based on poor model performance.

Unexplained models can be dangerous and costly in healthcare (N. D. Shah, Steyerberg, & Kent, 2018). With the current interest in DL methods—where interpretable or explainable models are not always possible—absolute clarity by developers and users is paramount for decision-making in medicine (i.e., diagnosis, prognosis) and must be understandable and conveyed to humans in plain language (Vellido, 2019). With the large movement from healthcare leaders and government to unblind features used in algorithmic testing (Topol, 2019) when there is a push for rush to market solutions (N. D. Shah et al., 2018), end user interpretability of all AI solution elements is paramount, based on their cognitive capacity, domain knowledge, and the explanation granularity (see Figure 3.9). The nuances in interpretability of AI model outputs, such as the differences between what is explainable, need comprehension by humans in natural language with easy to understand representations, as well as knowing what outputs are causal or prescriptive (Teredesai, Ahmad, Eckert, & Kumar, 2018).

ML algorithms do not guarantee the reflection of causal relationships or the actions to be taken based on an output as there could always exist unobserved causes responsible for associated variables (Lipton, 2016), and multiple decisions for a machine-driven prediction or suggestion for best practices. Utmost, personalized, intelligent medicine should be based on gold standard predictive solutions. The ability to understand AI algorithmic model interpretation, true performance, and to explain them, particularly in prediction, is in everyone's interest to ensure that prediction tools are as accurate as possible, most importantly for patient care (Glance, Dick, & Osler, 2018).

AI Solution Elements

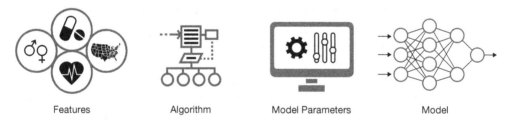

| Features | Algorithm | Model Parameters | Model |

User Interpretability

  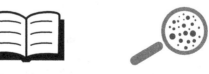

| Cognitive Capacity | Domain Knowledge | Explanation Granularity |

Figure 3.9 AI solution elements and user interpretability. Each component of an AI solution must be explainable for the solution to be explainable.

Source: Adapted from Lipton, Z. C. (2016). *The mythos of model interpretability* (pp. 96–100). Paper presented at ICML Workshop on Human Interpretability in Machine Learning, New York, NY; KenSci, Inc., 2018.

CONCLUSION

Like nurses, intelligent technologies learn through experience. In healthcare, superior human judgment in patient assessments, diagnosis, planning, interventions, and evaluations is paramount. Novel technologies, such as AI, that enhance these fundamentals of patient care through utilizing clinical support systems, as well as improving data management and day-to-day operations, are essential in modern medicine with rapid change in care and cost models, new treatments, and the need for high-quality, safe care to move patients successfully through the care continuum. In practice, the understanding that the domains of AI assist nurses with these processes and critical thinking, considering data source bias and equity and the need for ethics and policy, as well as governance and regulation, particularly with ML and DL processes, transparency, and understanding by healthcare professionals applying AI for expedited, precise clinical and administrative decision-making, are essential.

GLOSSARY

Algorithms: Sequential instructions and a set of well-constructed rules that ensure particular task completion.

Artificial Intelligence: The aptitude exhibited by smart machines broken down into perceiving, thinking, planning, learning, and the ability to manipulate objects.

Deep Learning: Cognitive intelligence algorithms that process Big Data inputs through hidden layer(s) of cells that adjust and connect to perform a task, and subsequently develop responses based on pattern recognition similar to how a human's brain responds to external stimuli.

Expert Systems: A technique that uses advanced computer programs to imitate the knowledge and reasoning capabilities of an expert in a particular discipline, with the endpoint being a tool that a layman can use to solve difficult or vague problems.

Machine Learning: A branch of AI where computer algorithms and programs improve automatically through experience concerning a class of tasks and performance measures.

Natural Language Processing: The automatic manipulation of natural, unstructured language, including text and speech, through algorithmic programming.

Predictive Analytics: A mathematic approach that uses statistical computations to analyze historical data from multiple sources to predict future events.

Reinforcement Learning: A type of behavioral model of machine learning technique that enables an agent to learn in an interactive environment by using feedback from its actions and experiences.

Supervised Learning: An algorithm that takes a known set of input data and known responses to the output data training model to generate reasonable predictions for the answers to new data.

Unsupervised Learning: An algorithm used to draw inferences from datasets consisting of input data only, without labeled responses to determine structure and patterns and uncover unobserved factors in unlabeled data.

THOUGHT-PROVOKING QUESTIONS

1. Understanding what AI is and what it is not, how will it inform the transformation of nursing roles, skills, and work environments?

2. Study the data types, purpose, and value in decision-making, Figure 3.2. Where in your care setting will nurses' decision-making be most impacted by predictive data? Why?

3. Considering the critical thinking and nursing process, in which phase(s) will AI enable a nurse to best capture patients' data for advanced analysis to predict an outcome? Once those data are collected, what are the next steps?

4. Name three ways in which NLP can help expedite care in your work setting.

5. Is it important to evaluate the outcomes of a machine or deep learning model? Explain your answer.

REFERENCES

Afzala, N., Mallipeddi, V. P., Sohn, S., Liu, H., Chaudhry, R., Scott, C. G., ... Arruda-Olson, A. M. (2018). Natural language processing of clinical notes for identification of critical limb ischemia. *International Journal of Medical Informatics*, *111*, 83–89. doi:10.1097/NCN.0b013e3181a91b58

Aiken, L. H., Cimiotti, J. P., Sloane, D. M., Smith, H. L., Flynn, L., & Neff, D. F. (2011). Effects of nurse staffing and nurse education on patient deaths in hospitals with different nurse work environments. *Medical Care*, *49*(12), 1047–1053. doi: 10.1097/MLR.0b013e3182330b6e

Alzantot, M. (2017). *Deep reinforcement learning demystified (Episode 0)*. Retrieved from https://medium.com/@m.alzantot/deep-reinforcement-learning-demystified-episode-0-2198c05a6124

Amarasingham, R. (2019, February 11). Innovative management: Social determinant networks to reduce excessive hospital utilization. Presentation at HIMSS19 Champions of Health Unite Global Conference and Exhibition, Orlando, FL. Retrieved from http://365.himss.org/sites/himss365/files/365/handouts/552514350/handout-NI3v3.pdf

American Medical Association. (2018). *Policy finder—Augmented intelligence*. Retrieved from https://policysearch.ama-assn.org/policyfinder/detail/augmented%20intelligence?uri=%2FAMADoc%2FHOD.xml-H-480.940.xml

Anderson, C., & Patterson, C. (2013). Collaborating on technology: A learning exchange between U.S. and U.K. nurses. *American Nurse Today*, *8*(11), SR5–SR6. Retrieved from https://www.americannursetoday.com/wp-content/uploads/2014/07/ant11-Technology-1107.pdf

Baratloo, A., Hosseini, M., Negida, A., & El Ashal, G. (2015). Part 1: Simple definition and calculation of accuracy, sensitivity and specificity. *Emergency*, *3*(2), 48–49. Retrieved from https://www.ncbi.nlm.nih.gov/pmc/articles/PMC4614595

Bari, A., Chaouchi, M., & Jung, T. (2017). *Predictive analytics for dummies* (2nd ed.). Hoboken, NJ: John Wiley & Sons.

Bates, D. W., Saria, S., Ohno-Machado, L., Shah, A., & Escobar, G. (2014). Big Data in health care: Using analytics to identify and manage high-risk and high-cost patients. *Health Affairs*, *33*(7), 1123–1131. doi:10.1377/hlthaff.2014.0041

Batra, G., Queirolo, A., & Santhanam, N. (2018, January). *Artificial Intelligence: The time to act is now*. Retrieved from https://www.mckinsey.com/industries/advanced-electronics/our-insights/artificial-intelligence-the-time-to-act-is-now

Bellman, R. E. (1978). *An introduction to Artificial Intelligence: Can computers think?* San Francisco, CA: Boyd & Fraser Publishing.

Bhatt, S. (2018). *5 things you need to know about reinforcement learning.* Retrieved from https://www.kdnuggets.com/2018/03/5-things-reinforcement-learning.html

Bogdanov, V. (2019, February 15). *8 thought-provoking cases of NLP and text mining use in business.* Retrieved from https://becominghuman.ai/8-thought-provoking -cases-of-nlp-and-text-mining-use-in-business-60bd8031c5b5

Breiman, L. (2001). Statistical modeling: The two cultures. *Statistical Science, 16*(3), 199–231. doi:10.1214/ss/1009213726

Bresnick, J. (2017). *Artificial Intelligence is altering healthcare, but not with "magic".* Retrieved from https://healthitanalytics.com/news/artificial-intelligence-is-altering-healthcare -but-not-with-magic

Buchanan, B. G. (2006). A (very) brief history of Artificial Intelligence. *AI Magazine, 26*(4), 53. doi:10.1609/aimag.v26i4.1848

Caffo, B., Leek, J., & Peng, R. (2016). *Machine learning—Class notes* [Google Docs Slides]. Retrieved from https://docs.google.com/presentation/d/1nbhPh8BjHHT_74rWYQKbyathfu qt5tF_z0z7KILpI8Q/edit#slide=id.g484b925ea_01

Carroll, W. M. (2019a, Winter). Artificial Intelligence, critical thinking and the nursing process. *Online Journal of Nursing Informatics, 23*(1). Retrieved from https://www .himss.org/library/artificial-intelligence-critical-thinking-and-nursing-process

Carroll, W. M. (2019b). The synthesis of nursing knowledge and predictive analytics. *Nursing Management, 50*(3), 15–17. doi:10.1097/01.NUMA.0000553503.78274.f7

Chen, J., Konnaris, A., Maier, J., Rangaswami, J. P., Ray, D., & Wachter, S. (2018). *Intelligent economies: AI's transformation of industries and society.* Retrieved from https://eiuper-spectives.economist.com/sites/default/files/EIU_Microsoft%20-%20Intelligent%20 Economies_AI%27s%20transformation%20of%20industries%20and%20society.pdf

Cipriano, P. F., & Hamer, S. (2013). Enabling the ordinary: More time to care. *American Nurse Today, 8*(11), 2–4. Retrieved from https://www.americannursetoday.com/ wp-content/uploads/2014/07/ant11-Technology-1107.pdf

Clipper, B., Batcheller, J., Thomaz, A. L., & Rozga, A. (2018). Artificial Intelligence and robotics: A nurse leader's primer. *Nurse Leader, 16*(6), 379–384. doi:10.1016/ j.mnl.2018.07.015

Cohen, J. K. (2018a, February). *How OSF HealthCare partners with community organizations to drive population health.* Retrieved from https://www.beckershospitalreview .com/data-analytics-precision-medicine/how-osf-healthcare-partners-with-community -organizations-to-drive-population-health.html

Cohen, J. K. (2018b, July 16). *12 healthcare use cases for natural language processing.* Retrieved from https://www.beckershospitalreview.com/artificial-intelligence/12 -healthcare-use-cases-for-natural-language-processing.html

Congress.gov. (2018). *National Security Commission on Artificial Intelligence Act of 2018.* Retrieved from https://www.congress.gov/bill/115th-congress/senate-bill/2806/ all-actions?overview=closed#tabs

Davenport, T. H., Hongsermeier, T. M., & Alba McCord, K. (2018). Using AI to improve electronic health records. *Harvard Business Review.* Retrieved from https://hbr .org/2018/12/using-ai-to-improve-electronic-health-records

Deng, L., & Yu, D. (2014). Deep learning: Methods and applications. *Foundations and Trends in Signal Processing, 7*(3/4), 197–387. doi:10.1561/2000000039

Downing, N. L., Bates, D. W., & Longhurst, C. A. (2018). Physician burnout in the electronic health record era: Are we ignoring the real cause? *Annals of Internal Medicine, 169*, 50–51. doi:10.7326/M18-0139

EchoNous. (2018). *The impact of AI on nursing: 5 key takeaways.* Retrieved from https:// echonous.com/en_us/discover/the-impact-of-ai-on-nursing-5-key-takeaways

The Economic Times. (n.d.). *Definition of 'data mining'*. Retrieved from https://economic times.indiatimes.com/definition/data-mining

The Economist. (2018). *AI, radiology and the future of work*. Retrieved from https://www .economist.com/leaders/2018/06/07/ai-radiology-and-the-future-of-work

Edwards, B. (2018, July 11). *Unlocking healthcare's Big Data with natural language processing*. Retrieved from https://www.chilmarkresearch.com/unlocking-healthcares -big-data-with-nlp-powered-ambient-and-augmented-intelligence

Elite Data Science. (n.d.). *Data science primer: Chapter 6: Model training*. Retrieved from https://elitedatascience.com/model-training

Elstein, A.S. (1999). Heuristics and biases: Selected errors in clinical reasoning. *Academic Medicine, 74*(7), 791–794. Retrieved from https://journals.lww.com/academicmedicine/ abstract/1999/07000/heuristics_and_biases__selected_errors_in_clinical.12.aspx

Erickson, B.J., Korfiatis, P., Akkus, Z., & Kline, T.L. (2017). Machine learning for medical imaging. *RadioGraphics, 37*, 505–515. doi:10.1148/rg.2017160130

Faggella, D. (2019). What is machine learning? *Emerj*. Retrieved from https://emerj .com/ai-glossary-terms/what-is-machine-learning

Frost & Sullivan. (2016). *From $600 M to $6 billion, Artificial Intelligence systems poised for dramatic market expansion in healthcare*. Retrieved from https://ww2.frost.com/ news/press-releases/600-m-6-billion-artificial-intelligence-systems-poised-dramatic -market-expansion-healthcare

Gartner. (2016). *2017 planning guide for data and analytics*. Retrieved from https://www .gartner.com/binaries/content/assets/events/keywords/catalyst/catus8/2017 _planning_guide_for_data_analytics.pdf

Gershgorn, D. (2018, September 6). *If AI is going to be the world's doctor, it needs better textbooks*. Retrieved from https://qz.com/1367177/if-ai-is-going-to-be-the -worlds-doctor-it-needs-better-textbooks/

Glance, L.G., Dick, A.W., & Osler, T.M. (2018). Risk prediction tools: The need for greater transparency. *Anesthesiology, 128*(2), 244–246. doi:10.1097/ALN.0000000000002021

Gn, C.K. (2018, August 31). *Artificial Intelligence: Definition, types, examples, technologies*. Retrieved from https://medium.com/@chethankumargn/artificial-intelligence -definition-types-examples-technologies-962ea75c7b9b

Gorry, A.G. (1984). Computer-assisted clinical decision making. In W.J. Clancey & E.H. Shortliffe (Eds.), *Readings in medical Artificial Intelligence—The first decade* (pp. 18–34). Reading, MA: Addison Wesley.

Gupta, V., & Birch, T. (2019). Using AI and natural language processing to uncover population social determinants of health factors. Presentation at HIMSS19 Champions of Health Unite Global Conference and Exhibition, Orlando, FL. Retrieved from http://365.himss.org/sites/himss365/files/365/handouts/552576703/handout-183.pdf

Hariharan, A. (2018, February 7). *How to use machine learning to predict the quality of wines*. Retrieved from https://medium.freecodecamp.org/using-machine-learning-to -predict-the-quality-of-wines-9e2e13d7480d

Hart, R.D. (2017, July 10). *If you're not a white male, Artificial Intelligence's use in healthcare could be dangerous*. Retrieved from https://qz.com/1023448/if-you re-not-a-white-male-artificial-intelligences-use-in-healthcare-could-be-dangerous/

Healthcare Information and Management Systems Society. (2018, December). *HIMSS Insights Series: Artificial intelligence* [eBook]. Retrieved from https://adobeindd.com/view/ publications/5c454ce9-309e-41bf-aed6-35f8f978e77c/kmye/publication-web-resources/ pdf/7.2_HIMSS_INSIGHTS_EBOOK_AI.pdf

Healthcare Information and Management Systems Society. (2019). *Unlocking the power of data analytics: New insights into key healthcare priorities and best practices* [Webinar]. Retrieved from https://www.himsslearn.org/unlocking-power-data -analytics-new-insights-key-healthcare-priorities-and-best-practices

Hodges, A. (2014). *Alan Turing: The enigma* (Rev. ed.). Princeton, NJ: Princeton University Press.

Holehouse, A. T. (n. d.). *Stanford machine learning: 01 and 02: Introduction, regression analysis, and gradient descent.* Retrieved from http://www.holehouse.org/mlclass/01_02_Introduction_regression_analysis_and_gr.html

Holzinger, A., Biemann, C., Pattichis, C. S., & Kell, D. B. (2017). *What do we need to build explainable AI systems for the medical domain?* Retrieved from https://arxiv.org/abs/1712.09923

Hurwitz, J., & Kirsch, D. (2018). *Machine learning for dummies—IBM limited edition.* Hoboken, NJ: John Wiley & Sons.

Hyun, S., Johnson, S. B., & Bakken, S. (2009). Exploring the ability of natural language processing to extract data from nursing narratives. *Computers, Informatics, Nursing, 27*(4), 215–225. doi:10.1097/NCN.0b013e3181a91b58

IBM Research. (n.d.). *AI and bias: Mitigating human bias in AI.* Retrieved from https://www.research.ibm.com/5-in-5/ai-and-bias

Institute of Medicine. (2010). *The future of nursing: Leading change, advancing health.* Washington, DC: National Academies Press.

Iriondo, R. (2019). *Differences between AI and machine learning and why it matters.* Retrieved from https://medium.com/datadriveninvestor/differences-between-ai-and-machine-learning-and-why-it-matters-1255b182fc6

Ismail, K. (2018). *AI vs. algorithms: What's the difference?* Retrieved from https://www.cmswire.com/information-management/ai-vs-algorithms-whats-the-difference

Jain, K. (2015). *Machine learning basics for a newbie: Machine learning applications.* Retrieved from https://www.analyticsvidhya.com/blog/2015/06/machine-learning-basics

Jensen, D. (2018). *GDPR deadline approaches: What is expected for compliance?* Retrieved from https://www.mastercontrol.com/gxp-lifeline/gdpr-deadline-approaches-what-is-expected-for-compliance

Johansen, M., & O'Brien, J. (2016). Decision making in nursing practice: A concept analysis. *Nursing Forum, 51*, 40–48. doi:10.1111/nuf.12119

Kiser, M. (2016, April 28). *An introduction to natural language processing.* Retrieved from https://medium.com/@mattkiser/an-introduction-to-natural-language-processing-e0e4d7fa2c1d

Klein, J. G. (2005). Five pitfalls in decisions about diagnosis and prescribing. *British Medical Journal, 330*, 781–784. doi:10.1136/bmj.330.7494.781

Kulikowski, C. A. (2015). An opening chapter of the first generation of Artificial Intelligence in medicine: The first Rutgers Aim workshop, June 1975. *Yearbook of Medical Informatics, 10*, 227–233. doi:10.15265/IY-2015-016

Kumar, A., Shukla, P., Sharan, A., & Mahindru, T. (2018). *National strategy for Artificial Intelligence.* Retrieved from http://niti.gov.in/writereaddata/files/document_publication/NationalStrategy-for-AI-Discussion-Paper.pdf

Kurzweil, R. (1990). *The age of intelligent machines.* Cambridge, MA: MIT Press.

Le, J. (2019). *A tour of the top 10 algorithms for machine learning newbies.* Retrieved from https://builtin.com/data-science/tour-top-10-algorithms-machine-learning-newbies

LeCun, Y., Bengio, Y., & Hinton, G. (2015). Deep learning. *Nature, 521*, 436–444. doi:10.1038/nature14539

Lipton, Z. C. (2016). *The mythos of model interpretability* (pp. 96–100). Paper presented at ICML Workshop on Human Interpretability in Machine Learning, New York, NY.

Liu, Y., Logan, B., Liu, N., Xu, Z., Tang, J., & Wang, Y. (2017). Deep reinforcement learning for dynamic treatment regimes on medical registry data. *Healthcare Informatics, 2017*, 380–385. doi:10.1109/ICHI.2017.45

Manyika, J., Lund, S., Chui, M., Bughin, J., Woetzel, J., Batra, P., . . . Sanghvi, S. (2017, November). *Jobs lost, jobs gained: What the future of work will mean for jobs, skills,*

and wages. Retrieved from https://www.mckinsey.com/featured-insights/future-of
-work/jobs-lost-jobs-gained-what-the-future-of-work-will-mean-for-jobs-skills
-and-wages

Marewski, J. N., & Gigerenzer, G. (2012). Heuristic decision making in medicine. *Dia-
logues in Clinical Neuroscience, 14*(1), 77–89. doi:https://www.ncbi.nlm.nih.gov/pmc/
articles/PMC3341653

Marino, M. V., Shabat, G., Gulotta, G., & Komorowski, A. L. (2018). From illusion
to reality: A brief history of robotic surgery. *Surgical Innovation, 25*(3), 291–296.
doi:10.1177/1553350618771417

Mastanduno, M. (2017). Machine learning 101: 5 easy steps for using it in healthcare.
Health Catalyst. Retrieved from https://www.healthcatalyst.com/learn-the-basics
-of-machine-learning-in-healthcare

MathWorks. (2019). *What is machine learning?: How it works, techniques & applications.*
Retrieved from https://www.mathworks.com/discovery/machine-learning.html

McGrane, C. (2018). *Health Tech Podcast: How AI is making humans the 'fundamental
thing in the Internet of things.'* Retrieved from https://www.geekwire.com/2018/
health-tech-podcast-ai-making-humans-fundamental-thing-internet-things

McLean, A. (2018). Nursing and Artificial Intelligence. *Canadian Journal of Nursing
Informatics, 13*(1). Retrieved from https://cjni.net/journal/?p=5355

Merriam-Webster. (n.d.). *Cybernetics.* Retrieved from https://www.merriam-webster
.com/dictionary/cybernetics

Miliard, M. (2018). HIMSS18: *Startup links community services with AI to improve social
determinant insights.* Retrieved from https://www.healthcareitnews.com/news/
himss18-startup-links-community-services-ai-improve-social-determinant-insights

Mitchell, T. (1997). *Machine learning.* Boston, MA: McGraw-Hill.

Mitchell, T. (2006). *The discipline of machine learning.* Retrieved from http://www.cs.cmu
.edu/~tom/pubs/MachineLearning.pdf

The MITRE Corporation. (2017). *Artificial Intelligence for health and health care.* Retrieved from https://www.healthit.gov/sites/default/files/jsr-17-task-002_aifor
healthandhealthcare12122017.pdf

Mulero, A. (2019). *FDA speeds up Artificial Intelligence approvals, review finds.* Retrieved from https://www.raps.org/news-and-articles/news-articles/2019/1/
fda-speeds-up-artificial-intelligence-approvals-r

Newell, A. (1982). *Intellectual issues in the history of Artificial Intelligence.* Pittsburg, PA:
Carnegie-Mellon University.

Ng, A. (2019). *AI for everyone. Coursera.* Retrieved from https://www.coursera.org/learn/
ai-for-everyone

Paul, R., & Heaslip, P. (1995). Critical thinking and intuitive nursing practice. *Journal of
Advanced Nursing, 22*, 40–47. doi:10.1046/j.1365-2648.1995.22010040.x

Pesapane, F., Codari, M., & Sardanelli, F. (2018). Artificial Intelligence in medical imaging: Threat or opportunity? Radiologists again at the forefront of innovation in
medicine. *European Radiology Experimental, 2*(1), 35. doi:10.1186/s41747-018-0061-6

Pieces Tech. (2018a). *Client success: Early warning system can save lives* [Slide Set].

Pieces Tech. (2018b, April). *Pieces Tech solution overview* [Slide Set].

Pieces Tech. (2019, February 13). *Pieces Tech and Ensocare join forces to address patients' social determinants of health.* Retrieved from https://piecestech.com/
pieces-tech-ensocare-join-forces-address-patients-social-determinants-health

Piper, K. (2019, April 4). Winner of Turing Test award—The AI breakthrough that
won the "Nobel Prize of computing". *Vox.* Retrieved from https://www.vox.com/
future-perfect/2019/4/4/18294978/ai-turing-award-neural-networks

Polson, N., & Scott, J. (2018). *AIQ: How Artificial Intelligence works and how we can harness
its power for a better world.* New York, NY: Penguin Random House.

Press, G. (2016). *A very short history of Artificial Intelligence (AI)*. Retrieved from https://www
.forbes.com/sites/gilpress/2016/12/30/a-very-short-history-of-artificial-intelligence
-ai/#ff4f98a6fba2

Qureshi, I. (2018, October 26). *Healthcare data scientists: 6 steps for utilizing your data analysts*. Retrieved from https://www.healthcatalyst.com/insights/
healthcare-data-scientists-steps-leveraging-data-analysts

Reed, J. (2016). *Gaining business insight for clinical trials—Text analytics for a data driven approach*. Retrieved from https://www.prismeforum.org/wp-content/uploads/2015/12/
PRISME_Linguamatics_TextAnalytics_ClinicalData-Jane-Reed.pdf

Risling, T. (2018). *Why AI needs nursing*. Retrieved from http://policyoptions.irpp.org/
magazines/february-2018/why-ai-needs-nursing

Rowe, J. (2019). *Health policy analysts call for more rigorous AI monitoring*. Retrieved from
https://www.healthcareitnews.com/ai-powered-healthcare/health-policy-analysts
-call-more-rigorous-ai-monitoring?

Russell, S., & Norvig, P. (Eds.). (2010). *Artificial Intelligence: A modern approach* (3rd ed.).
New York, NY: Prentice Hall.

Seif, G. (2019, June). *An easy introduction to natural language processing: Using computers to understand human language*. Retrieved from https://builtin.com/data-science/
easy-introduction-natural-language-processing

Sensmeier, J. (2017). Harnessing the power of Artificial Intelligence. *Nursing Management*,
48(11), 14–19. doi:10.1097/01.NUMA.0000526062.69220.41

Shah, N. D., Steyerberg, E. W., & Kent, D. M. (2018). Big Data and predictive analytics:
Recalibrating expectations. *Journal of the American Medical Association*, *320*(1), 27–28.
doi:10.1001/jama.2018.5602

Shah, S., & Joffe, R. (2018). *How AI is evolving in diagnostic imaging*. Retrieved from https://
www.diagnosticimaging.com/automation/how-ai-evolving-diagnostic-imaging

Silver, D., Hubert, T., Schrittwieser, J., Antonoglou, I., Lai, M., Guez, A., ... Lillicrap, T.
(2018). A general reinforcement learning algorithm that masters chess, shogi, and
Go through self-play. *Science*, *362*(6419), 1140–1144. doi:10.1126/science.aar6404

Simpson, R. (2012). Technology enables value-based nursing. *Nursing Administration Quarterly*, *36*(1), 85–87. doi:10.1097/NAQ.0b013e318237b7b4

Skiba, D. (2017). Augmented intelligence and nursing. *Nursing Education Perspectives*,
38(2), 108–109. doi:10.1097/01.NEP.0000000000000124

Smith, A. (2018, February). What's the difference between machine learning, AI, and
NLP? *Quora*. Retrieved from https://www.quora.com/Whats-the-difference-between
-machine-learning-AI-and-NLP

Smith, C., McGuire, B., Huang, T., & Yang, G. (2006). *History of computing CSEP 590A:
The history of Artificial Intelligence*. Seattle, WA: University of Washington.

Stanford Medicine. (2018). *Stanford Medicine 2018 health trends report—The democratization of health care*. Retrieved from https://med.stanford.edu/content/dam/sm/
school/documents/Health-Trends-Report/Stanford-Medicine-Health-Trends
-Report-2018.pdf

Stanford Medicine. (2019). *Equity, AI inclusion in health care with AI technology*. Retrieved
from https://med.stanford.edu/presence/initiatives/ai.html

Teredesai, A., Ahmad, M. A., Eckert, C., & Kumar, V. (2018). *Explainable models for healthcare
AI*. Retrieved from https://learning.acm.org/techtalks/healthcareai

Tocco, S. (2013, July 11). Human factors engineering can improve patient safety.
American Nurse Today. Retrieved from https://www.americannursetoday.com/
human-factors-engineering-can-improve-patient-safety

Topaz, M., Dowding, D., Lei, V. J., Zisberg, A., Bowles, K. H., & Zhou, L. (2015). Using
natural language processing to automatically identify wound information in narrative
clinical notes: Application development and testing. *Proceedings of the Home Healthcare*,

Hospice, and Information Technology Conference (H3IT), 2, 22. Retrieved from https://h3it.org/_static/assets/docs/proceedings/H3IT-2015-Proceedings.pdf

Topaz, M., & Pruinelli, L. (2017). Big Data and nursing: Implications for the future. *Studies in Health Technology and Informatics*, 232, 165–171. doi:10.3233/978-1-61499-738-2-165

Topol, E. (2019). *Deep medicine: How Artificial Intelligence can make healthcare human again.* New York, NY: Basic Books.

Torres, B. G. (2016). The true father of Artificial Intelligence. *OpenMind*. Retrieved from https://www.bbvaopenmind.com/en/technology/artificial-intelligence/the-true-father-of-artificial-intelligence

Turing, A. M. (1950). Computing machinery and intelligence. *Mind*, 59, 433–460. doi:10.1093/mind/LIX.236.433

U.S. Food and Drug Administration. (2019a). *De Novo classification request.* Retrieved from https://www.fda.gov/MedicalDevices/DeviceRegulationandGuidance/HowtoMarketYourDevice/PremarketSubmissions/ucm462775.htm

U.S. Food and Drug Administration. (2019b). *FDA statement: Statement from FDA Commissioner Scott Gottlieb, M.D., and Jeff Shuren, M.D., Director of the Center for Devices and Radiological Health, on a record year for device innovation.* Retrieved from https://www.fda.gov/NewsEvents/Newsroom/PressAnnouncements/ucm629917.htm

van Stralen, K. J., Stel, V. S., Reitsma, J. B., Dekker, F. W., Zoccali, C., & Jager, K. J. (2009). Diagnostic methods I: Sensitivity, specificity, and other measures of accuracy. *Kidney International*, 75(12), 1257–1263. doi:10.1038/ki.2009.92

Vellido, A. (2019). Societal issues concerning the application of Artificial Intelligence in medicine. *Kidney Diseases*, 5, 11–17. doi:10.1159/000492428

VEX Robotics. (n.d.). *What is robotics?* Retrieved from https://curriculum.vexrobotics.com/curriculum/intro-to-robotics/what-is-robotics.html

Vyborny, C., and Giger, M. (1994). Computer vision and artificial intelligence in mammography. *American Journal of Roentgenology, (162)*3, p. 699.

World Information. (n.d.). 1980s: *Artificial Intelligence (AI)—From lab to life—Expert systems.* Retrieved from http://world-information.org/wio/infostructure/100437611663/100438659445/print?ic=100446326244

Zhou, L. (2018). *How to build a better machine learning pipeline.* Retrieved from https://www.datanami.com/2018/09/05/how-to-build-a-better-machine-learning-pipeline

Zhou, L., Plasek, J. M., Mahoney, L. M., Karipineni, N., Chang, F., Yan, X., … Rocha, R. A. (2011). Using Medical Text Extraction, Reasoning and Mapping System (MTERMS) to process medication information in outpatient clinical notes. *AMIA Annual Symposium Proceedings*, 2011, 1639–1648. Retrieved from https://www.ncbi.nlm.nih.gov/pmc/articles/PMC3243163/

ADDITIONAL RESOURCES

Business Dictionary. (2019). *Definition—Statistical inference.* Retrieved from http://www.businessdictionary.com/definition/statistical-inference.html

Schulman, J. (2016). *Deep reinforcement learning.* Retrieved from http://learning.mpi-sws.org/mlss2016/slides/2016-MLSS-RL.pdf

Shortliffe, E. H. (1992). The adolescence of AI in Medicine: Will the field come of age in the '90s? *Artificial Intelligence in Medicine*, 5, 93–106. doi:10.1016/0933-3657(93)90011-q

4

Virtual Reality, Augmented Reality, and Mixed Reality

BARBARA FICARRA

CHAPTER OBJECTIVES

- Define Virtual Reality (VR), Augmented Reality (AR), and Mixed Reality (MR).
- Identify how applied immersive technologies are utilized in patient care.
- Summarize how VR/AR/MR is applied to medical, nursing, and patient education.

CONTENTS

INTRODUCTION

The global healthcare market for Virtual Reality (VR), Mixed Reality (MR), and Augmented Reality (AR), or VR/AR/MR, known collectively as "immersive technologies," is a multibillion-dollar industry (Bellini et al., 2016; Global Industries Analysts, Inc., 2019; Market Watch, 2019; Zion Market Research, 2019). These promising technologies continue to gain momentum as a powerful diagnostic tool and aid in the treatment and management of patients in the clinical setting. VR, a fully immersive three-dimensional (3D) simulation, shuts out the real world and transposes the patient to "somewhere else" (Curtin, 2017). It is used as distraction therapy and a tool to help decrease pain and anxiety for the pediatric patient (Wolitzky, Fivush, Zimand, Hodges, & Rothbaum, 2005). It is useful for the obstetric patient and the adult patient for the treatment of wounds. It is further used to assist in the treatment of mental health conditions such as depression, anxiety, phobias, posttraumatic stress disorder (PTSD), and severe pain in burn victims (Maples-Keller, Bunnell, Kim, & Rothbaum, 2017). VR/AR/MR used in the clinical setting, hospitals, and health systems can help clinicians better engage with their patients, elevate the patient experience, and provide more personalized care (Deloitte, 2018). Furthermore, these innovative and emerging technologies are applied in the educational setting. Nursing students and medical students enhance their learning practice and training by harnessing the power of these technologies. It allows students an immersive experience and permits students an unrestricted practice of procedures. Immersion is described as a deep absorption, being immersed in something. For example, a real or artificial environment or an activity.

Moreover, MR encompasses the spectrum from AR to VR, blending the physical and digital worlds to produce new environments where physical and digital objects coexist and interact in real time to educate and train nursing and medical students and healthcare professionals (S. Kos, Microsoft, personal communication, May 31, 2019).

This chapter provides a brief historical overview of immersive technologies and summarizes how they are applied in nursing and medical education. It explores how nursing and medical students engage with these technologies in the educational setting. It further explores how it is used in the clinical setting for training to improve patient safety. It examines how these advanced innovations lead to a new course for nurse educators, researchers, and informaticists. Due to the evolution of these immersive technologies, this chapter offers details to expand and transform the role of the nurse leader in nursing education, nursing researchers, and nurse informaticists. It provides key takeaways to pursue or expand a career in healthcare technology. It delves into ways the nurse educator and researcher can harness these technologies to support learners in attaining their goals. Additionally, it examines how it is used for training simulation by the healthcare professional. Furthermore, this chapter explores the various ways in which VR/AR/MR are used in the healthcare setting, specifically exploring how it is utilized with the pediatric population from emergency department visits to inpatient visits. It addresses the nurse's role in VR/AR/MR use and how nurses engage their patients to help distract them and to help manage their pain and anxiety. Lastly, this chapter explores thought-provoking questions to engage the reader.

In this chapter, VR/AR/MR use focuses on academic applications for educators and the training of nurses and doctors, as well as to inform patient care and the pediatric population. Immersive technologies are poised to transform and impact nursing and medical education as well as patient care. Excitement abounds as it continues to create strides and makes its way into the hands of educators, students, patients, and care teams. In addition, emerging technologies are capable of transforming the trajectory in academics by creating opportunities for nurse and medical educators, researchers, and informaticists. Also, pursuant to this innovative technology, it has the potential to expand and pivot the role of nurses and doctors in the technology space in the healthcare arena.

VIRTUAL REALITY, AUGMENTED REALITY, AND MIXED REALITY: DEFINITIONS

Virtual Reality (VR) is technology designed to immerse and transport the user into a "virtual world" (Table 4.1). VR is an intervention with an immersive and interactive, 3D display that excludes the external (real-world) environment (Chan, Foster, Sambell, & Leong, 2018) but resembles real-life interactions (Chirico, Ferrise, Cordella, & Gaggioli, 2018). It is a computer-simulated environment (Haluck, 2000) accessed through a head-mounted display (HMD; A. Li, Montaño, Chen, & Gold, 2011). It allows users to be fully immersed in the experience. VR is multisensory (Chirico et al., 2018), allows the user to perceive of being "present" in the environment (Chirico et al., 2018), and is a completely

Table 4.1 Type of Immersive Technology, Definition, and Market Products Used for Patient Care, and Medical, Nursing, and Patient Education

Type of Reality	Definition	Market Products
Virtual	VR is a completely immersed digital experience, providing a realistic simulation of a three-dimensional environment that is experienced and controlled by movement of the body.	FundamentalVR Osso VR Pocket Nurse Sharecare YOU
Augmented	Layers digital, interactive objects on top of the physical environment without the ability to manipulate based on environmental awareness.	Immersive Touch Proprio MAI SentiAR Proximie
Mixed	Encompasses the spectrum from AR to VR, blending the physical and digital worlds to produce new environments where physical and digital objects coexist and interact in real time.	Microsoft HoloLens Microsoft HoloLens2 Magic Leap VimedixAR With HoloLens

AR, Augmented Reality; VR, Virtual Reality.
Source: S. Kos, personal communication, May 31, 2019.

immersed digital experience, providing a realistic simulation of a 3D environment that is experienced and controlled by movement of the body (S. Kos, Microsoft, personal communication, May 31, 2019).

Augmented Reality (AR) is technology that allows the user to see the real-world right in front of him or her, with objects overplayed on the digital content. It takes the visual information and superimposes it on the physical environment. A good example of this technology is the app-based game Pokémon Go.

AR layers digital, interactive objects on top of the physical environment without the ability to manipulate based on environmental awareness (S. Kos, Microsoft, personal communication, May 31, 2019).

Mixed Reality (MR) is technology that is similar to AR, as it combines both VR and AR. MR integrates both the simulated and real-world environments to create an experience where real-world and virtual-world objects interact with each other in real time. An example is Microsoft's HoloLens (The Franklin Institute, n.d.-b). It uses advanced sensors for gesture recognition and spatial awareness (Cook, Jones, Raghavan, & Saif, 2017). MR encompasses the spectrum from AR to VR, blending physical and digital worlds to produce new environments where objects coexist and interact in real time (S. Kos, Microsoft, personal communication, May 31, 2019).

VIRTUAL, AUGMENTED, AND MIXED REALITY IN HEALTHCARE: YESTERDAY AND TODAY

Immersive technologies of today build upon ideas that date back to the 1800s, almost to the very beginning of practical photography. The term "virtual reality," however, was first used in the mid-1980s when Jaron Lanier, founder of VPL Research, began to develop the gear, including goggles and gloves, needed to experience what he called "Virtual Reality" (The Franklin Institute, n.d.-a). Lanier's research and engineering contributed a number of products to the blooming VR industry (Lowood, n.d.).

Today, VR is being applied in the healthcare setting, from clinical practice to nursing and medical education. The research from over 10 years ago to the present suggests and supports the effectiveness of emerging technologies for patient care and educational and clinical training. Historically, the cost of VR was quite expensive. A featured article published on the American Psychological Association's website states that 10 years ago, the cost to set up VR was US$30,000, and the equipment was large and bulky (Weir, 2018). The technology has improved over the years and also become more cost-effective. VR technology is now streamlined, according to Brandon Birckhead, MD (B. Birckhead, personal communication, February 8, 2019), and today the cost is about US$200.00 for a headset, or HMD. Cedars-Sinai Medical Center is one of the leading institutions using VR for their patients, with the vast majority of users being the adult population. Immersive technology is used for pain management and to help decrease anxiety. At Cedars-Sinai, of the patients who have trialed it, VR has had some impact on pain, regardless of pain type, and patients are able to tolerate it well (B. Birckhead, personal communication, February 8, 2019). The Microsoft HoloLens has been used by a number of academic and healthcare institutions; its second iteration, HoloLens 2, will be available the end of 2019 at a price of US$3,500 (S. Kos, Microsoft, personal communication, May 31, 2019).

HEALTHCARE LANDSCAPE

The healthcare landscape is changing and pivoting, and the health industry is beginning to engage and operationalize these innovative technologies to help improve patients' lives, patient care and outcomes, and to educate and train nurses and doctors. Technology is revolutionizing healthcare and patients are more connected in their care. Not only is technology getting smarter, but patients today are becoming savvier to emerging technologies and their health. Patients are intrinsically remarkably smart—they know their own bodies and context of their lives—and no one has a bigger interest in their own health (Topol, 2015, p. 8). Nurses recognize this and the phenomena of patients remaining silent without questioning their treatments, care plans, medications, activities of daily living, and nutrition has passed to a state where they are now determined to speak up and ask questions, requiring a partnership with care teams. Trust and transparency are critical to patients. Increasingly, the nurse–patient relationship bond and communication is strengthening, and to keep up with inquisitive and savvier patients, nurses require targeted training in order to provide the best, highest quality care possible and to enhance the patient's healthcare journey through improved experience. Immersive technology aids in patient engagement, enabling patients to be empowered, proactive, and engaged in their care. It is essential that nurses and hospital leaders leverage technology to keep the patient at the center of care, and, while doing so, always keep the human connection alive. Nursing is the intersection of art, science, and technology. Humanizing care in the most empathizing manner will never be lost in the quest to expand innovative technology.

THERAPEUTIC USE OF VR/AR/MR: FOCUS ON THE PEDIATRIC POPULATION

Immersive Technology for Reducing Anxiety and Pain

Today immersive technology is not only for entertainment; it is also making its way to the bedside into "clinical areas" (A. Li et al., 2011). Providing quality patient care and making the hospital experience more tolerable for children in particular is a priority in healthcare. The healthcare ecosystem is transforming; to stay current with the modern digital culture, many companies are developing emerging technologies to improve pediatric patient care. VR, AR, and MR are making strides in healthcare. This revolutionary technology helps foster improved patient experience and quality of care by focusing on the needs of the pediatric patient. This patient population requires special attention, care, and treatment, and addressing the psychosocial needs of the pediatric patient is paramount. Clinical settings can be very scary and stressful for children and provoke anxiety. To help ease pain and uneasiness through therapeutic distraction, immersive technology is impacting and enhancing patient-centered care.

A visit to a pediatric emergency department (PED) requiring specialized medical procedures can be psychologically traumatizing and emotionally threatening, and a scary place for pediatric patients (DeClercq et al., 2018; Lerwick, 2016), and anxiety among pediatric patients can be significant (Heilbrunn et al., 2014).

A type of anxiety experienced in a PED is known as situational or state anxiety (both known as SA; Heilbrunn et al., 2014; Nager, Mahrer, & Gold, 2010), and it may be difficult to detect and treat in children (Heilbrunn et al., 2014; MacLaren et al., 2009). The American Academy of Pediatrics (AAP) posits that healthcare professionals have a responsibility to address anxiety in the PED and create more favorable environmental conditions for pediatric patients (Fein, Zempsky, & Cravero, J. P.; Committee on Pediatric Emergency Medicine and Section on Anesthesiology and Pain Medicine, 2012; Heilbrunn et al., 2014) to meet the imperative that the needs of a child are met and that healthcare professionals, the family, and the child collaborate to optimize their care (Dudley et al., 2015). Trust, communication, respect, empathy, emotional support, and empowerment are vital for the pediatric patient and his or her family members. Monitoring and treating pediatric patients require an extra level of care in their healthcare process (Lerwick, 2016). Nurses and physicians must understand the anxiety and trauma in pediatric patients with regard to receiving medical care, and treatment is imperative to quality of care and positive outcomes. It is essential for nurses and physicians to take time to explain to the pediatric patient the reason for the treatment in a developmentally appropriate manner to help decrease his or her anxiety. If anxiety increases, the child may feel helplessness, which results in lack of cooperation. If the child feels anxious, clinical-patient trust is broken (Lerwick, 2016). Nurses and physicians must establish trust and empower the pediatric patient.

When children present to the PED, they are often subjected to procedures that can cause anxiety and pain. Controlling stress, anxiety, and pain for children is a critical component of emergency medical care (Fein et al., 2012). To manage the children's pain and anxiety, aside from pharmacologic interventions, distraction is a simple and effective technique that redirects children's attention away from noxious stimuli (Koller & Goldman, 2012). Distraction can be in the form of support from a child life specialist, television, books, video games, bubbles, kaleidoscopes, music, images on a wall, or sitting on a parent's lap (Trottier, Ali, Le May, & Gravel, 2015). In keeping up with the digital ethos in healthcare, VR, AR, and MR can play a new, impactful role in pediatric therapeutic distraction.

In addition to humanizing patient care with competent, dedicated, and empathetic nurses and physicians to help alleviate pain, anxiety, and stress in the pediatric patient, novel technological interventions can prove beneficial. Immersive technology, specifically VR, may help to provide a helpful psychological and physiological environment to expedite rehabilitation for pediatric patients suffering from chronic (Won et al., 2017), procedural, and acute pain. VR has been shown to be a distractor to help alleviate pain and anxiety associated with invasive medical procedures, such as venipuncture (Won et al., 2017), lumbar punctures, and bone marrow aspirations (Gershon, Zimand, Lemos, Olasov Rothbaum, & Hodges, 2003).

VIRTUAL REALITY

VR can be used to make the pediatric patient more familiar, comfortable, and calm with procedures (Won et al., 2017). This innovative technology may prove beneficial because children are increasingly comfortable with interacting with technology, such as playing video games. In modern society, children and adolescents are surrounded by technology and are immersed in a digital environment (Reid Chassiakos et al., 2016). Eighty-four percent of teens say they have or have access to a game console at home, and 90% play video games of some kind (Anderson & Jiang, 2018), with 67% of Americans ages 2 and older playing video games on at least one type of device, with over half of these playing across multiple platforms such as computers, game consoles, or cellphones (The NPD Group, 2018). Engaging pediatric patients in clinical settings with an **immersive experience** where they become profoundly absorbed and entrenched in the experience is possible, and the ability to distract from aversive interventional stimuli is possible. Like video games, VR has the potential to engage children in an imaginary world (Gershon, Zimand, Pickering, Rothbaum, & Hodges, 2004), creating an illusion (Steele et al., 2003) that the pediatric patient using this technology is immersed and entrenched in a virtual environment, where a 3D world can be seen, and the patient can engage and interact by moving his or her head and neck, much like playing currently marketed technology-based games.

Pediatric patients engaged in VR have reported that the distraction was a pleasant experience. It succeeded at distracting patients and has proven successful at lessening procedural pain and distress related to needle-related procedures and intravenous (IV) placement (Won et al., 2017), with VR significantly reducing anxiety and acute procedural pain (Gold & Mahrer, 2018). According to Chan et al. (2019), VR intervention was effective and safe in children from 4 to 11 years old undergoing venipuncture or IV cannulation. It showed a decrease in anxiety, distress, and needle pain; despite the study having limitations. Additionally, a randomized controlled trial found that, out of a group of 143 children, those who wore a VR headset during blood draws reported experiencing less pain and anxiety than patients who did not (Gold & Mahrer, 2018). Currently, at Stanford Children's Health/Lucile Packard Children's Hospital, AR and VR are used to improve patient care and expand the patient experience. At Stanford Children's Health/Lucile Packard Children's Hospital CHARIOT program in Palo Alto, California, VR/AR are utilized for children with needle phobias and those enduring medical procedures or undergoing surgery, anesthesia, physical therapy, or occupational therapy (T. Caruso, personal communication, June 19, 2019), proving tolerable and beneficial in therapeutic treatment (Case Study 4.1).

CASE STUDY 4.1

PEDIATRIC NEEDLE PHOBIA ADDRESSED WITH VR

Anxiety and fear, such as fear of needles, or needle phobia, is a prevalent issue in children. According to Yuan, Rodriguez, Caruso, and Tsui (2017), needle phobia can progress to a debilitating mental illness. Needle phobias can also lead to patient's avoidance of invasive medical care. Success in using a novel nonpharmacological method via a provider-controlled Virtual Reality (PCVR) headset that displays a customized game for a pediatric patient prior to surgery has been used in a pediatric clinical setting.

A 10-year-old anxious pediatric patient with a history of needle phobia presented for bilateral orchiopexy under planned intravenous (IV) induction of anesthesia. Prior to preoperative anesthesia, the pediatric patient was fitted with a customized Samsung

(continued)

CASE STUDY 4.1 (*continued*)

Gear VR headset equipped with a Samsung Galaxy S8 smartphone. Permission was granted by parents prior to utilizing this system. Developed by the Stanford Child-hood Anxiety Reduction through Innovation and Technology (CHARIOT) program specifically for children undergoing minor procedures, the PCVR was loaded with a game called Spaceburgers™. This technology immerses patients in outer space, where they are instructed to "zap" space objects. A button on the side of the VR headset (or hand controller) allows care teams to temporarily increase the frequency of objects flying toward the patient (in "turbo mode"). Immediately prior to the needle punc-ture procedure, turbo mode was initiated on the VR device, and the nurse was able to successfully place a 22-gauge IV catheter with no interruption or patient discomfort. This enhanced VR technology improved the pediatric patient experience because it distracted the patient and drew the attention away from the fear and the anticipation of needle-induced pain. The patient conveyed satisfaction with the VR experience, noting the IV insertion was the least painful needle encounter and the best experience at a hospital. The patient's mother also expressed that she would recommend VR for other anxious children (Yuan et al., 2017).

Therapeutic VR is a unique and promising new modality with the potential to treat serious and debilitating medical conditions by delivering a low-risk, nonpharmacological intervention (J. Sackman, personal communication, May 22, 2019). As mentioned, VR may help lower stress and anxiety and, by becoming fully immersed in VR, it may also help manage postsurgical pain for children. Postsurgical rehabilitation in the pediatric patient can be extremely painful; often, pharmacological analgesics are not able to control the pain (Steele et al., 2003) and nonpharmacological interventions such as VR, which creates the illusion that the patient is immersed in a virtual world, can be used to reduce postsurgical pain and thus improve patient outcomes (Steele et al., 2003). The following case study explores how the use of VR served as a nonpharmacological analgesic for children following surgery (Steele et al., 2003; Case Study 4.2).

VR IN THE PEDIATRIC EMERGENCY DEPARTMENT: A NURSE'S EXPERIENCE

Orange Regional Medical Center in Middletown, New York, utilizes VR as part of the patient experience for pediatric patients who are identified as requiring a reduction in pain and anxiety, as well as an aid for distraction. "VR is one tool in the tool-kit," said Michelle Ferguson, MS, CCLS, CEIM, CPST, Child Life Program Coordinator (M. Ferguson, personal communication, April 3, 2019), and it offers psychosocial support to help minimize trauma, she further explained. At Orange Regional Medical Center, the VR devices are supplied by Applied VR. Ferguson explained that it is the nurse who assesses the child and identifies whether or not the child will benefit from VR use (M. Ferguson, personal communication, April 3, 2019).

"VR is a good distraction for painful procedures or scary situations," said Melissa Zuber, RN, Emergency Department nurse at the same hospital (M. Zuber, personal communication, April 3, 2019). "VR gives [patients] something

CASE STUDY 4.2

VIRTUAL REALITY AS A PEDIATRIC PAIN MODULATION TECHNIQUE

One study reveals that VR use as a nonpharmacological analgesia for the pediatric patient undergoing a single-event multilevel surgery (SEMLS) post-procedure is effective in reducing pain (Steele et al., 2003). A 16-year-old male with cerebral palsy at the Women's and Children's Hospital in Adelaide, Australia, participated in a VR immersion post-procedure study. Permission was granted by the patient and parents prior to VR therapy. For each of nine physiotherapy sessions, the patient spent half of the session, approximately 10 minutes, using VR with pharmacological analgesics. The other half of the physiotherapy session, the patient used only pharmacologic analgesics. The patient, using the FACES scale, supported the hypothesis that VR may have an analgesic effect. Additionally, the parents also noted a decrease in the patient's anxiety with an increase in motivation. The parent also noted that because her son was more relaxed, she felt less anxious. Interestingly, the study states that the therapist had to work harder to engage the patient during active treatment during VR use because the patient was completely immersed in the game (Steele et al., 2003).

else to focus on … if we see a child that we're having a hard time consoling or needs a little distracting and we want to make the experience a bit more bearable, we will call the child life specialist and let her know what we need" (M. Zuber, personal communication, April 3, 2019). While it is the child life specialist who is called to assist with the technology, it is the nurse who identifies the need. "From my experience, I can tell you we see immediate results and most kids are pretty intrigued when they see it," she said (M. Zuber, personal communication, April 3, 2019). The immediate results she is referring to is the decrease in anxiety and pain. The children are usually happy because they are thinking they are actually playing the game and it is "fun time" (M. Zuber, personal communication, April 3, 2019; Figure 4.1).

M. Zuber (personal communication, 2019) explains that VR is used for children who need blood drawn, IV insertions, and intermuscular (IM) injections. The contraindications include children with a history of motion sickness and seizures. VR is not used on any child under 4 years of age. Ferguson stated it is not to be used more than 30 minutes at a time, but there is no limit on the frequency. Typically, she said it is used from 5 to 15 minutes. The "Bear Blast – Dodge Ball with Bears" is a popular game with the children. According to M. Zuber (personal communication, April 3, 2019), each device costs approximately between US$3,500.00 and US$5,000.00, and while they are successful with this innovative technology, it will never replace the child life specialist's role in assisting with pediatric patients. "Our role is a partnership," she said. "The nurses are well informed, and they identify the need; together we collaborate and utilize VR for those children who we think it will help make the hospital experience more bearable. VR will never replace us, 'it's a great asset to the skill sets,' and it is 'one tool in the tool-kit.'"

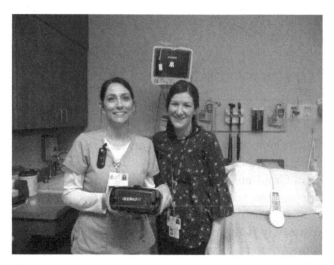

Figure 4.1 Melissa Zuber, RN, and Michelle Ferguson, MS, CCLS, CEIM, CPST, Child Life Program Coordinator, with VR equipment at Orange Regional Hospital.
Source: Courtesy of Barbara Ficarra, April 3, 2019.

The detailed VR protocol to reduce pain and anxiety and aid distraction in the PED is as follows (M. Ferguson, personal communication, April 3, 2019):

1. Identify the appropriate patient to use VR. The nurse will assess age, risk factors, symptoms, and patient's presenting complaint, and then validate that the patient does not have a history of seizures, is not presently nauseous. and does not have headaches.
2. Assess pain, anxiety level, and blood pressure. The nurse will have the patient complete a quantitative survey and case report form to identify pre and post pain and anxiety levels after using VR.
3. Obtain equipment from a Child Life Specialist. The nurse will use the VR tool kit binder to check out the equipment and ensure proper documentation using the patient's sticker.
4. Review use of VR with patient and proper use of device for providers. The nurse will refer to the AppliedVR "How to Administer AppliedVR Treatment" handout (Exhibit 4.1).
5. Launch VR experience. The nurse will show the patient the focus dial, reaffirm he or she must remain seated or in bed, and inform the patient that he or she can take off headset at any time.
6. Monitor the patient's experience. The nurse will monitor the patient's experience and equipment safety.
7. Reassess the patient's pain, anxiety level, and blood pressure after use of AppliedVR and procedure completion. The nurse will use the case report form found in the binder to record the patient's level of pain, anxiety, and blood pressure post experience.
8. Return device to the proper area after the patient's use. The nurse will document check-in time in the binder and identify the nurse who returns the device back.
9. Clean device per manufacturer's recommendations. The nurse or emergency technician will wipe down the headset with a sanitary agent, and wipe down the lens with lens wipe, then let dry 2 minutes before use with the next patient.

EXHIBIT 4.1
EXAMPLE OF A PEDIATRIC INPATIENT SURGICAL WORKFLOW USING VIRTUAL REALITY

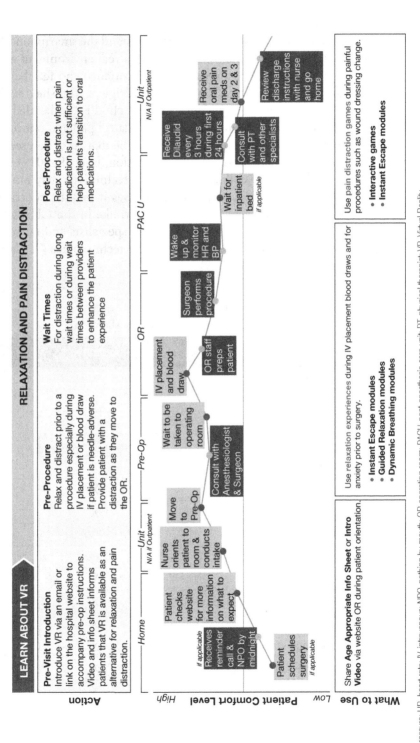

BP, blood pressure; HR, heart rate; IV, intravenous; NPO, nothing by mouth; OR, operating room; PACU, post-anesthesia care unit; PT, physical therapist; VR, Virtual Reality.

Source: Reproduced with permission from AppliedVR. (n.d.). Inpatient workflow for VR [Slide set].

It is also noted in the protocol that if the patient experiences any harmful side effects, remove the device immediately, reassess the patient, and report any events to the charge nurse.

AUGMENTED REALITY

The simplest way to describe AR is to understand the smartphone app Pokémon Go. It superimposes visual information on a real environment and is akin to a hologram in space. AR is an ideal tool for patients who fear being in the fully immersive experience that VR provides (Rodriguez, Munshey, & Caruso, 2018). AR is a fully immersive experience where a child is "embedded in game play" that can reduce anxiety; in some cases, pediatric patients opt for AR over VR because through the headset children describe that "they can see me, and I can see them" (T. Caruso, personal communication, June 19, 2019). It is important to note that for many children, immersive technology may not be useful as a therapeutic intervention, and in certain cases it may be contraindicated (see Table 4.2). For this reason, it is crucial that, like in the CHARIOT program, interprofessional teams including child life specialists and nurses assess which patients are good candidates for immersive technologies (T. Caruso, personal communication, June 19, 2019).

Table 4.2 VR and AR Indications and Contraindications

Condition/Procedure	Indicated	Contraindicated
Bone marrow aspiration	X	
Chest tube removal	X	
Claustrophobia		X
Dizziness		X
History of seizures[a]		X
IV cannulation	X	
Lumbar puncture	X	
Motion sickness[a]		X
Nausea		X
Occupational therapy	X	
Orthopedic procedure-pin removal	X	
Physical therapy	X	
Posttraumatic stress disorder	X	
Surgery: Pre- and postoperative	X	
Venipuncture	X	
Wound dressing change	X	

AR, Augmented Reality; IV, intravenous; VR, Virtual Reality.

[a]*Source:* Data from Yuan, C., Rodriguez, S., Caruso, T., & Tsui, J. (2017). Provider-controlled virtual reality experience may adjust for cognitive load during vascular access in pediatric patients. *Canadian Journal of Anesthesia, 64*(12), 1275–1276. doi:10.1007/s12630-017-0962-5

Nurses may wonder why a patient needs to use immersive technology goggles when a patient can simply use his or her own device to watch an inline video that may distract him or her or play a game on a smart device. In fact, with immersion with VR/AR/MR, by wearing goggles, the mind perceives it as another place, and therefore the patient won't look around and lose focus because wearing the goggles fully immerses the experience instead of focusing on an external environment (T. Caruso, personal communication, June 19, 2019; Case Study 4.3).

The priority of any hospital is to provide quality patient care. Caring for and treating children is specialized and requires empathetic nurses and doctors—ones who humanize healthcare. Emerging technologies aid in the transformation of healthcare. VR, AR, and MR are promising emerging technologies that assist in the treatment and management of patients experiencing procedural and acute pain. The applications of VR/AR/MR are applied to children undergoing medical and painful procedures; it is used as a distraction to help decrease their pain and anxiety. This technology is not new, but the growth is slow and steady in the healthcare sector, and it has the potential to proliferate.

CASE STUDY 4.3

AUGMENTED REALITY FOR INTRAVENOUS ACCESS IN AN AUTISTIC CHILD WITH DIFFICULT VENOUS ACCESS

This case study illustrates the successful use of AR glasses in the perioperative care of a pediatric patient with autism who refused VR glasses. An anxious, autistic, morbidly obese (BMI 57), 11-year-old child with multiple poor intravenous (IV) experiences was presented for esophagogastroduodenoscopy (EGD). Two novel nonpharmacological techniques to reduce anxiety were discussed with the patient and the family: VR and AR glasses. The child declined the VR glasses because he wanted to "see what is going on" and opted for AR glasses as they allowed for partial immersion while still being able to see his surroundings. Upon wearing the AR glasses, interactive cartoon holograms, named Ben and Jenny, projected in front of the patient through a Microsoft HoloLens, which encompasses AR and MR. The experience was mirrored onto a tablet that allowed providers to know exactly what was in the patient's field of view. Once the patient said, "IV Prep," Ben and Jenny began discussing the IV cannulation process in an interactive and playful fashion. Aspects such as access sites, indications, and needle pain–reducing tactics were discussed with the patient prior to the procedure. To enhance engagement, the child brought his fingers together in front of the screen to fire virtual paintballs at anything in his vision. At this point, the IV was performed. Throughout the process, the patient remained engaged with the glasses while periodically looking at the needle. At no point did the child appear anxious. After successful cannulation, the mother was extremely satisfied, and the child described the experience as "the best IV I've ever gotten."

Source: Rodriguez, S., Munshey, F., & Caruso, T. J. (2018). Augmented reality for intravenous access in an autistic child with difficult access. Pediatric Anesthesia, 28(6), 569–570. doi:10.1111/pan.13395. Reproduced with permission from Wiley.

Robust literature review suggests that VR/AR/MR are safe and effective to help eliminate pain and anxiety from medical procedures during an emergency department (ED) or hospital admission. Recent studies and clinical trials support research from over 10 years ago. Technology has become more affordable, and nurses and doctors have access to a promising and engaging intervention for acute and chronic pain in the pediatric patient. It is important to note that while technology has the power to help transform healthcare, the role of nurses and doctors is critical. It is their expertise, skill, and empathy that will always be of utmost importance.

THE REDESIGN OF NURSING, MEDICAL, AND PATIENT EDUCATION WITH IMMERSIVE TECHNOLOGIES

Emerging technologies have ventured into healthcare education. A review of the literature suggests a slow and steady growth of VR, AR, and MR use in the classroom, for training and in the clinical setting. Examination of the literature reveals significant benefits for students using digital technology. Using immersive technologies for nursing and medical education is changing the landscape and culture in education. Applying immersive technologies to the classroom and training centers pivots the educational learning style, and it brings realism to the clinical setting for nursing and medical students. It is making strides in training nurses and doctors. The clinical setting is a controlled and risk-free environment (Jenson & Forsyth, 2012), which allows for unlimited practice of procedures (Jenson & Forsyth, 2012). Utilizing VR in the classrooms provides a safe environment to reflect and learn (Fertleman et al., 2018). This type of technology has existed for decades; however, with recent advances in technology, it is now beginning to infiltrate into education and healthcare. It is an exciting and emerging field (Fertleman et al., 2018). By harnessing the powers of this innovative technology in the classroom and clinical setting, it not only changes the trajectory of the education and training but offers new opportunities for nurses in the technology space in the healthcare arena.

These distinctive immersive technologies have the potential to move education from its dependence on lectures and textbooks to experiential learning (Helsel, 1992). An exciting frontier, these innovative technologies pose new and thrilling opportunities for nurse educators, professors, medical instructors, nurse researchers, and nurse informaticists. Healthcare professionals within these specialties have the opportunity to become actively involved in the implementation and progress of VR/AR/MR. Moreover, these advanced technologies have the potential to serve as a powerful educational tool for patients.

Traditionally, nursing and medical students have mounds of books (Pappano, 2018), lectures, notes, lecture recordings, educational videos, memory aids, and clinical rotations. However, the conventional style of learning is changing. Digital technology has transformed the way people live, work, and play, and it is altering the way students learn. Millennials, or Gen Y, ages 23 to 38 years old (Dimock & Dimock, 2019), are technologically savvy (Rogers, 2018). It is reported that 74% of millennials feel that technology makes their lives simpler and 54% feel that new technology brings them closer to family and friends (Rogers, 2018). The rich experience of VR is alluring to millennials, and they are two times more likely to purchase a VR headset than their generational peers. VR heightens the sense of memory and this is appealing to millennials (Rogers, 2018). Thus, immersive technology in the classroom is a prudent step. Lectures are becoming obsolete in some institutions (Farber, 2018), and innovative technologies have made their way into the classroom setting and the clinical setting for training. VR/AR/MR are beginning to take center stage in the educational arena. While these immersive technologies are appealing to students and are instrumental in education and training, a question raised is will this technology replace textbooks in the academic setting? The notion that VR/AR/MR will contribute to the demise of textbooks is unfounded. Textbooks and e-books continue to be used in medical and nursing schools. For example, The University of Illinois College of Medicine has a robust list of books students need outlined on their website (The University of Illinois College of Medicine, 2019) and Georgetown University School of Nursing and Health Studies requires textbooks for their students (Georgetown University School of Nursing and Health Studies, 2019). The aforementioned are only two simple examples, but a significant one to illustrate the importance of textbooks in the classroom. Therefore, immersive technologies are becoming part of the educational toolkit, not a complete replacement. Some universities may have made lectures obsolete, but textbooks continue to have their place in education along with advanced technologies. In keeping up with the millennial generation, nursing and medical students use these technology applications as part of their learning curriculum. Students gain access to the virtual world through visualization, simulation, and training skills. Moreover, hospitals and health systems have begun to implement this technology to train their staff. According to The University of Nebraska Medical Center's website, the US$118.9 million facility is poised to transform healthcare education, and propel the training of nurses, doctors, and allied health professionals into the next generation with emerging VR and AR (Burbach, 2017). This technology has a potential to boom in the marketplace. The global healthcare market for VR, AR, and MR is a multibillion-dollar industry (Chen, 2016; Global Industries Analysts, Inc., 2019; Market Watch, 2019; Zion Market Research, 2019), and by 2025 it is expected to reach US$5.1 billion (Brightman, 2016; CISION-PRN Newswire, 2017; ReportBuyer, 2017). VR/AR is expected to lead the U.S. market (Brightman, 2016).

With the potential to flourish and expand the market, this technology is gaining momentum in educating students and clinicians. VR can provide a rich, engaging, and interactive educational experience (Mantovani, Castelnuovo, Gaggioli, & Riva, 2003). Students learn by doing, and VR can contribute to an increase in motivation and raise interest in the curriculum (Mantovani et al., 2003).

These advanced technologies enable nursing and medical students to be transported into a **3D simulation** of real-life patient experience (Jenson & Forsyth, 2012). This fully immersive 3D virtual experience allows students to explore the accurate anatomical model of the human body, its organs, and their natural function (Sharecare, n.d.), and VR has the structure to provide students the opportunity to learn by interactive role-play (Lippincott Nursing Education, 2017). Further VR learning tools for students include the virtual dissection table (Anatomage Table) and virtual simulation (Lateef, 2010) or Virtual Reality simulation (VRS), which simulates real-life procedures and other real-life nursing experiences. Furthermore, MR/AR applications, such as Microsoft's HoloLens, immerse students into hologram experience to improve their learning experience.

Educational Redesign: Changing the Culture

At Harvard University, traditional lectures, for the most part, are obsolete. Students are opting to learn the course work at home instead of spending hours in a lecture. By learning the course material on their own time and often with videos, students are spending less time in an auditorium and are learning the course content at home, which they then apply in mandatory small group sessions (Farber, 2018). Vermont Medical School has also done away with lectures. According to an interview with the dean of the school, on NPR, lectures are not good at engaging students and "not the best way to accumulate the skills needed to become a scientist or a physician" (Cornish & Gringlas, 2017). VR/AR/MR are hands-on learning. If lectures are not good at engaging students, perhaps these advanced, immersive technologies are a better way for students to learn. Educational institutions call for innovation and are prompted to meet educational needs in a new way (Murray, 2013).

In order to keep up with the digital era, the classroom is changing to meet the technology needs of the students. Educators are responding powerfully to the notion of VR/AR/MR as part of the nursing and medical curriculum. A review of the literature suggests that students do not want to be in a classroom listening to lectures. They want to be hands-on, active, and engaged in the process (Mantovani et al., 2003). VR/AR/MR is an engaging experience. These innovative technologies foster and enhance the learning process and promote an environment that can be tailored to individual learning and performance style (Mantovani et al., 2003).

The Robert Wood Johnson Foundation; the Center to Champion Nursing in America; and the U.S. Department of Labor, Employment and Training Administration commissioned *Blowing Open the Bottleneck: Designing New Approaches to Increase Nurse Education Capacity*, a White Paper (Joynt & Kimball, 2008) that encourages innovative thinking and multi-stakeholder teams to design and implement creative ways to educate nurses. Nurse educators are rethinking how nurses are educated and they are looking at strategies that are more effective and efficient (Joynt & Kimball, 2008). A literature review supports the posing threat of a significant nursing shortage over the next 20 years, and the pressure to educate more nurses in a more disciplined and efficient manner is mounting (Joynt & Kimball, 2008). However, the educational infrastructure is failing to keep pace with the growing number of nursing students enrolled. There is a shortage of nurse faculty and clinical education sites (Joynt & Kimball, 2008). The nursing profession has its challenges, but depleting nursing education can have devastating effects. Nurses are the backbone to healthcare, and the most trusted profession (American Hospital Association, 2019); redesigning nursing education is a prudent and mandatory step. The mission of nurses, outlined by the American Nurses Association, is to improve health for all (American Nurses Association, n.d.), and it is a priority of the World Health Organization (WHO, 2019). One miniscule, but important aspect to improve health for all incorporates a robust educational system for nurses. This allows nurses to learn and acquire cutting-edge skills in order to provide quality care and treatment of patients. Education is critical and it has a significant impact on the competencies and knowledge of the nurse clinician (American Association of Colleges of Nursing, 2019). Nursing educational curriculums need resuscitating and a redesign. Quality patient-centered care, patient safety, empathy, compassion, patient and family education, and leadership are the heart and core of what nurses value, and nurse educators have an instrumental role in helping them fulfill it.

With innovation and design thinking, technology can help revive a progressive yet challenging profession. **Design thinking** is defined as a human-centered approach to tackling new problems through exploring new ideas with alternatives that haven't existed before. What do humans need? What makes life more enjoyable or easier? What makes technology practical and useful? (Brown, 2009). A significant redesign in nursing education using immersive technology is needed to prepare highly competent and better-equipped nurses to meet the demands of healthcare, and to improve quality and safety. By exploring a new way to tackle the issue of education, using a divergent approach may help change the culture. What is very intriguing about Joynt and Kimball's White Paper is the fact that the White Paper is over 10 years old. Today, emerging technologies are creating strides in healthcare. However, it may still be in the infancy stage in many settings. As the White Paper points out, clinical education is the most expensive part of nursing education, and cost becomes an issue. However, the traditional model of nursing education makes inadequate use of time for both faculty and student.

Technology is a prudent choice and the natural next step for the learning process. In this digital world, student learning is enhanced via technology. Technology can improve productivity, accelerate learning, and increase student engagement and motivation (U.S. Department of Education, n.d.). The National League for Nursing—Institute for Simulation and Technology encourages nurse educators to "stay-up-to-date" on simulation, innovation, informatics, and telehealth (National League for Nursing, n.d.-a), and encourage educators to prepare students for advances in technology in healthcare. **Telehealth** is defined as the use of electronic information and telecommunication technologies to support long-distance clinical healthcare, patient and professional health–related education, public health, and health administration. Technologies include video conferencing, the Internet, store-and-forward imaging, streaming media, and terrestrial and wireless communications (U.S. Department of Health and Human Services, 2019).

The National League for Nursing (NLN) champions simulation technology in nursing education. As stated on their website, simulation "is rapidly gaining common ground as a standard teaching strategy" (NLN, n.d.-b). The virtual world, vSim, facilitates learning through unfolding real-world, evidence-based scenarios (Laerdal Medical AS, 2015). The NLN is a proponent of technology, and encourages the use of vSim, and collaborates with Wolters Kluwer Health and Laerdal Medical on the development of vSim. vSim is a comprehensive learning tool that brings simulation technology to the students (Wolters Kluwer: Lippincott Nursing Education, 2018). However, vSim is not a virtual immersive experience. It utilizes avatars with online interaction and helps students prepare for practice, but it is not the 3D immersive experience elicited by VR/AR/MR. This opens the doors for nurse educators to bring 3D emerging technologies to the attention of the NLN and in the classrooms.

Simulation

There are different types of simulation. First, what is simulation? Simulation is the imitation of a process or system. Secondly, simulation is not all equal. In nursing education and medical education, the types of simulators available are varied and can be categorized as "standardized patients, partial-task trainers, mannequins (high-fidelity patient simulators), screen-based computer simulators, and virtual-reality simulators" (Chakravarthy et al., 2011). Lastly, the type of technology varies by colleges and universities and in the clinical setting.

To further explain simulation, one example is the standardized patient, human patient simulation using mannequins (low-fidelity and high-fidelity), and it is found at Yale University, Yale School of Nursing. The website explains "labs are equipped with video and audio recording systems and sessions include a faculty or peer review recordings made during the session in order to enhance learning outcomes" (Yale School of Nursing. n.d., "Current Capabilities"). As previously discussed, there is the virtual and computer base simulations (Laerdal Medical AS, 2015; NLN, 2015), encouraged by the NLN. Simulation is an evaluation tool, as well as a teaching strategy, and it is cost-effective compared to other tools (S. Li, n.d.). However, these types of simulations are significantly different from AR/MR simulation that is used to educate and train healthcare professionals. Moreover, while cost may be a consideration, keeping up with cutting-edge emerging technology cannot be overlooked. Emerging technologies, such as immersive VR, "could become commonplace in nursing education" (Kilmon, Brown, Ghosh, & Mikitiuk, 2010 , p. 315).

The robust literature review reveals that while there are some educational institutions and hospital settings using immersive technologies for nursing education, it does not appear commonplace to date. However, an emerging paradigm for educational training AR/MR simulation can reshape learning and is used in some hospitals. CAE Healthcare provides innovative training solutions using simulation to help improve patient safety (CAE Healthcare Videos, 2018). Dr. Chad Epp, President, Society for Simulation in Health Care, said in a YouTube video, "What we see in this generation of learners is that they come to the classroom with a different set of skills, eager to interact with technology, eager to be immersed in their learning environment" (CAE Healthcare Videos, 2018). Students want an immersive experience. This **3D technology** is used in universities and hospitals (CAE Healthcare Videos, 2018) and it is a learning tool for doctors, nurses, military medics, and first responders (Bloomberg, n.d.). "For centuries, people were relying on textbooks and dissection and plastic models of the heart and in the span of twenty years, we've seen that augmented reality on a 3D screen, and now what HoloLens added is another layer," said Dr. Robert Amyot, President, CAE Healthcare, in a YouTube video. He added, "You're not looking at augmented reality on a 3D screen, it's there, standing in mid-air and now we can see these finite details" (CAE Healthcare Videos, 2018).

Virtual, Augmented, and Mixed Reality in Nursing Education

To meet the needs in this technology era, there are some institutions redesigning education by incorporating VR/AR/MR into the nursing school curriculum. Immersive technologies (VR/AR/MR) are forging ahead in education. Students are learning by interacting with technology; they are learning by interacting with holograms. Mixed Reality (MR) technology such as HoloLens enables users to interact with holograms in the same ways that they interact with other physical objects (S. Kos, Microsoft, personal communication, May 31, 2019). By interacting with physical objects, students have a better understanding. Nursing students at the University of Canberra in Australia are using the HoloLens to learn patient assessments with a virtual holographic patient (Canberra, 2017). "This is a hologram that's right in front of you, it's life size," said Mark Christian, Global Director of Immersive Learning, Pearson in the YouTube video (Canberra, 2017). It's a visual medium, it's about interacting with patients, interacting with people; it has real potential, he explained (Canberra, 2017). Redesigning nursing education with technology allows students to be involved in a virtual learning environment, a life-like 3D immersive experience. VR/AR/MR can aid between theory and practice for nursing students. It bridges the gap in education and paves the way to make learning more efficient and fun. It allows students to live the experience; as it engages the students, it can help maximize learning (Maresky et al., 2019). VR engages the students and maximizes learning. VR has also been associated as a tool for teaching empathy, and it may enhance empathy (Louie et al., 2018). However, further research is needed. In a PubMed search, the results for VR as a tool for nurses to learn empathy is scarce. This is an area where research can further be explored.

As emerging and versatile technologies, VR/AR/MR have the potential to transform health profession education. In a study published in the *Journal of Medical Internet Research*, posted January 22, 2019, findings showed that VR may have the ability to improve skills and postintervention knowledge as compared to the traditional style of education "or other types of digital education, such as online or offline digital education" (Kyaw et al., 2019, "Results").

The number of institutions, both academic and clinical, applying immersive technologies are reasonable, but, as previously mentioned, not commonplace. In addition to Canberra University, Penn State University offers the Penn State IMEX Lab to its health profession students, and offers biological (life) science students the opportunity to visualize, navigate, and explore how the body works using VR and Sharecare YOU by Sharecare Inc. (Sharecare, n.d.). The 3D immersive experience takes students inside the human body. Using Oculus Rift or HTC Vive, this VR technology gives students and staff a virtual view where they can "step inside" the body. The author utilized and practiced with the Sharecare YOU VR device and chose to be transported into the heart and colon. An immersive experience with clear details and accurate physiology, it simulates diseases and medical conditions. Experiencing a healthy body to a disease state, the VR immersive experience is a teaching tool with movement with head and body allowed the experience "to come to life" (Penn State University Libraries, 2019).

First year medical students at the University of California San Francisco use VR to learn anatomy. Students can "pull the muscles apart" on the virtual cadaver; they can then build and rebuild it. "VR will enhance the students' understanding of the arrangement of the body," said Derek Harmon, PhD, USCF Assistant Professor of Anatomy in the YouTube video (Baker, 2017). He further adds, "In virtual reality they can go from skin level all the way down to the bones and take every single layer off as they go and see the relationships, how they're stacked up, how they're aligned and when they get to the bones they can repeat it, almost like a puzzle and put all the pieces right back on there all the way back out to the skin." The immersive experience can be transported inside the body and move through it (Baker, 2017). VR used to learn anatomy is not only for medical students. Nursing students could benefit greatly from this technology to learn anatomy. This is another area that opens the doors for nurse educators. They have the power to harness this 3D technology and help deploy it in colleges and universities for anatomy class.

The Yale University medical and nursing schools use technology in their classrooms. The medical school uses AR to learn anatomy and nurses use the Microsoft HoloLens to provide a viral experience on high fidelity patient simulation mannequins. "Students at West Coast University's Los Angeles campus, the largest nursing school in the country uses the HoloLens for education," said Kos in an email interview (S. Kos, Microsoft, personal communication, May 31, 2019). "It has been among the first in the country to implement HoloLens into their learning experience, and they have seen amazing results. WCU anatomy students are scoring a full letter grade higher when learning in augmented reality vs. a traditional textbook," he said. The University of Canberra also uses the HoloLens to educate students. Kos further explained that "Pearson, an education publishing and assessment service for schools and corporations, has developed HoloPatient which provides standardized patient experiences for medical education at Texas Tech University" (S. Kos, Microsoft, personal communication, May 31, 2019; LaFreniere, 2017; San Diego State University, 2017). One of the unique features of the HoloLens is the ability for students to engage and interact with the holograms by using hand gestures and word commands (Craig & Georgieva, 2017).

At Western University in Pomona, California, The J and K Virtual Reality Learning Center (VRLC) offers innovative and cutting-edge technology to deliver a deeply engaging learning experience for their students in health sciences. Disciplines include nursing, osteopathic medicine, pharmacy, health sciences, veterinary medicine, optometry, dental medicine, podiatry, and biomedical science. Students learn in a virtual environment. From using VR immersion technology using Oculus Rift to take a virtual tour of the human body to using the Anatomage Virtual Dissection Table, to two zSpace and the Stanford anatomical models on a tablet, these technologies are engaging active learners to ultimately lead to enhanced patient care (Gaudiosi, 2015; Western University of Health Sciences, n.d.).

In the *Journal of Internet Medical Research*, "Virtual Reality for Health Professions Education: Systematic Review and Meta-Analysis by the Digital Health Education Collaboration" (Kyaw et al., 2019), a total of 31 studies with 2,407 participants and meta-analysis of eight studies suggests that VR slightly improves postintervention knowledge scores compared with the traditional style of learning or other types of digital education such as online or offline digital education. Another meta-analysis of four studies suggests that VR improves cognitive skills of health professionals compared with traditional learning (Kyaw et al., 2019). While this offers positive results, the authors suggest further research is needed to evaluate the effectiveness of VR technology on outcomes such as satisfaction, cost-effectiveness, attitudes, and clinical practice or behavior change (Kyaw et al., 2019). The benefits are wide; however, a vast literature review reveals the importance of further studies. There are drawbacks; some users have experienced dizziness or nausea while using VR (Dyer, Swartzlander, & Gugliucci, 2018).

Patient Education

To humanize care, as well as empower and engage patients, healthcare is leveraging immersive technology. To transform the patient experience and educate patients, hospitals are using VR for patient education. This is an exciting sector and the potential for VR to educate patients is powerful. However, after an extensive literature search, information is lacking in this area. Perhaps VR is only in the infancy stage for patient education.

One example of a hospital using VR to educate patients is Boston Children's Hospital. Boston Children's Hospital partnered with Klick Health to bring Health Voyager to their patients. Patients (and their parents) are able to visualize their disease (Klick Health, 2018). Health Voyager is VR technology that provides the patient with a 3D tour of an endoscopy or colonoscopy (Heath, 2018). The patients see exactly what the clinicians see during the procedure. Patients use their own smartphones; after scanning a bar code, it allows them access to their 3D tour. They will either use a VR headset or clip-on glasses or Google Cardboard (Heath, 2018). This technology is interactive, and it allows clinicians to educate their patients about their medical conditions (Heath, 2018). Stanford Children's Health is another example of a hospital using VR for patient education. Pediatric cardiologists at Stanford Children's Health—Lucile Packard Children's Hospital Stanford use VR immersive technology to educate patients with complex congenital heart defects by explaining this difficult medical condition in a 3D virtual, engaging way (Stanford Children's Health, 2017). Cognitant is a health technology that aims to help educate patients with 3D virtual technology. Patients wear a VR headset such as the Oculus Go and their medical condition and treatment options are explained via technology. Their first VR/smartphone content is currently in the pilot stage and it is set to help women make the right choice about their contraception (Kent, 2019).

Immersive technology, 3D VR, can pivot patient education. Engaging patients with technology enables them to have an interactive experience and can make learning difficult medical conditions fun and engaging. This is an area that further needs to be developed. VR, a powerful tool, is only skimming the patient education surface.

Benefits to Medical Education

VR/AR/MR is useful in the educational setting. The benefits and goals of using VR/AR/MR in nursing and medical education include an immersive and engaging experience (see Table 4.3), positively enhancing students' learning experience (Madathil et al., 2017), and students acquiring new skills and knowledge (Zhu, Hadadgar, Masiello, & Zary, 2014). Furthermore, students perceive improvement in learning outcomes (Madathil et al., 2017), which improves skill coordination (Guze, 2015) and strengthens cognitive-psychomotor abilities (Zhu et al., 2014). It may also help improve postintervention skills and knowledge (Kyaw et al., 2019; Zhu et al., 2014), enhance perceptual variation (Guze, 2015), improve decision-making and psychomotor skills (Guze, 2015), improve grades (S. Kos, Microsoft, personal communication, May 31, 2019), and prolong learning retention and shorten their learning curve (Zhu et al., 2014). Research supports the impact VR has with

Table 4.3 Benefits of Immersive Technologies in Nursing Education and Medical Education

Benefits of Immersive Technologies	Source
Immersive and engaging experience that positively enhances the students' learning experience	Madathil et al. (2017)
Students acquire new skills and knowledge	Zhu et al. (2014)
Students perceive improvement in learning outcomes	Madathil et al. (2017)
Improves skill coordination	Guze (2015)
Strengthens cognitive-psychomotor abilities	Zhu et al. (2014)
Helps to improve postintervention skills and knowledge	Kyaw et al. (2019); Zhu et al., 2014
Enhances perceptual variation	Guze (2015)
Improves decision-making and psychomotor skills	Guze (2015)
Improve grades	Kos (personal communication, 2019)
Prolongs learning retention and shortens the students' learning curve	Zhu et al. (2014)

teaching medical and health profession students in developing empathy (Dyer et al., 2018). Additional benefits of this technology include learning team training, and practicing for critical or rare events (Guze, 2015), as well as helping to improve surgeons' skills (Piromchai, Avery, Laopaiboon, Kennedy, & O'Leary, 2015; Seymour et al., 2002).

VR/AR/MR is making its way into the hands of nurses, doctors, and patients. It is important to note that it is not common to find a technology set in the electronic medical record (EMR). "Presently, there's no order set," said Brandon Birckhead, MD, project scientist for VR clinical trials at Cedars-Sinai Medical Center, Los Angeles, California (B. Birckhead, personal communication, February 8, 2019). "Currently, most activities are through clinical trials," he said. Birckhead further explained that Cedars-Sinai receives calls from other departments outside of the clinical trial arena to implement VR in other departments. Pain medicine services, nurses, integrative medicine services, and spiritual services will call and request VR services. "This would be off clinical trial, but we try to help when we can," he said. He further explained, "the best way to get implemented into a hospital level is if there was an EMR order set." By having VR in the EMR, "someone on the team, a virtualist or staff member with particular skills and knowledge in this area, could go and round like other services. I could see VR becoming a pillar of technology—a digital health pillar that is used for pain reduction, mental health and education for patients and providers. This is another tool in the toolkit" (B. Birckhead, personal communication, February 8, 2019).

EXPANDING THE NURSE'S ROLE WITH THE USE OF VR/AR/MR

A 2017 study by Wolters Kluwer and the NLN found that nursing programs using technology are projected to change over the next 5 years (Wolters Kluwer: Lippincott Nursing Education, n.d.). It reports that 65% of programs are using visual simulation and about half are expected to use VR within 5 years. According to the survey, 10% of nursing programs are presently utilizing VR (Wolters Kluwer: Lippincott Nursing Education, n.d.). This is good news for nurse innovators because as emerging technologies continue to expand, nurses can harness the power of VR/AR/MR to help educate students, train nurses in the clinical setting, and educate patients.

Adapting VR/AR/MR in the academic and clinical setting will continue to flourish, and applying these emerging technologies provides a safe environment to learn and grow. The vast research supports the use of these emerging technologies in the classroom for nursing and medical education. To fully utilize this useful training tool for nurses and doctors, there is a need for educators versed in technology and science. The advancement of technology in healthcare leads to greater opportunities. Staff nurses, nurse informaticists, nurse educators, nurse researchers, nurse scientists, nurse investigators, and nursing professors have the potential to expand their career path into the technology sector, specifically immersive technologies. They have an exciting opportunity to spearhead and benchmark themselves in the technology arena. As immersive technologies continue to expand, there will be a need for nurses and medical educators with a strong base of clinical expertise to spearhead projects using VR/AR/MR. In 1992, Helsel wrote that "virtual reality holds much promise for education," and that "educators need to become involved now to plan for VR's future development, planning, and use with students" (Helsel, 1992, p. 42). Not only is there an opportunity for nurse educators, nurse informaticists, and nurse researchers to become actively engaged in immersive technology for nursing education, but patient education is an area where nursing expertise is needed to design, implement, and use VR with patients. To help educate patients to make informed decisions and to inform patients on disease and prevention, VR can be utilized to enhance their learning. There is a significant opportunity to spearhead patient education using technology.

It is critical for nurse educators, researchers, and informaticists to align themselves with significant stakeholders in the healthcare technology ecosystem. They should create a strong online presence and engage frequently with key players. Also, they should attend meet-ups, conferences, networking events, industry events, and collaborate and communicate. As these professionals design a benchmark for themselves and look for familiar skill sets with industry experts, windows of opportunities abound. Create a "one-page" document that highlights your strengths and establish yourself as a technology go-to expert. Design and create a technology council at your institution. Contact nursing organizations to develop or expand technology innovation. Develop a business plan and identify how emerging technologies can enhance the learning experience, challenge the learning process, aid in patient education, and improve quality care and outcomes. Emerging technologies for patient education are for the most part unexplored areas. As nurse leaders, challenge the status quo and move forward into the technology area to transform the healthcare landscape. Also, as Birckhead alluded to, VR is not part of the EMR. This is an opportunity for nurse informaticists to spearhead projects to move this area forward. Additionally, the opportunity for nurses to lead clinical trials has great promise. Interested nurses ought to contact leading institutions utilizing these emerging and immersive technologies and begin to expand technology at colleges, universities, and health systems for projects to implement VR/AR/MR in the classroom, clinical setting, and with patient education.

CONCLUSION

While the use of immersive technologies for nursing and medical students becomes gradually implemented, it is not commonplace. However, with the projected market, it has the potential to flourish. Forward-thinking nursing professionals have a wide range of opportunities to spearhead and cultivate projects to implement VR/AR/MR in the classroom, clinical setting, and with patient education.

Emerging technologies aid in the transformation of healthcare. VR/AR/MR are promising technologies that offer significant opportunities to continue to revolutionize healthcare. Leveraging these technologies in institutions for students and clinicians is invaluable. Nursing students and medical students harness the power of these technologies to enhance their learning practice. It allows students an immersive experience and permits students an unrestricted practice of procedures. These innovative emerging technologies are implemented in the clinical setting and are the hallmark of clinician training. These immersive technologies can help advance nursing education, and these advanced innovations lead to a new course for nurse educators, researchers, professors, and informaticists, which may improve the learning experience (Allcoat & von Mühlenen, 2018). The use of technology in education complements learning; it should not be a replacement for face-to-face learning or textbooks, but instead be used as a supplemental tool. "Educators must still focus on the [principles] of teaching, not on the specific technologies" (Guze, 2015, p. 267). There are robust benefits to using VR/AR/MR but there are drawbacks such as nausea and dizziness.

It is important to note that immersive technology alone is not the only solution for improved patient outcomes and quality care. While it can help promote learning and help improve patient care, healthcare is about the patient. It is about nurses and doctors engaging in an honest, empathetic, and compassionate manner with their patients. In *Well*, Sandro Galea writes, "Compassion is what makes humans human. It reminds us of our shared vulnerability to the broader conditions that shape health" (Galea, 2019, p. 85). Nurses have enormous power to help shape health by leveraging their education and bringing their knowledge, skills, and expertise to their patients. Whether treating and caring for patients in the hospital, educating patients and their families, or leading in the public setting as health educators, nurses have a powerful influence to help shape healthcare and set parameters for immersive technologies. Whether educating nursing students or training seasoned nurses in a clinical setting to keep them abreast of the newest and updated policies and procedures, immersive technology is at the cornerstone. What may change the educational shift is not the idea of technology, but the idea to create and cultivate another realm in the classroom and clinical arena to ultimately improve patient care and foster health for all. Nurses will be at the forefront of keeping a delicate balance between technology and the human experience alive. Nurse leaders have the power to harness innovative technologies and catapult patient care into the connected generation; and to establish design parameters that ignite and invigorate a vibrant healthcare ecosystem.

GLOSSARY

3D Simulation: Shuts out the real world and transposes the patient to "somewhere else"; it is used as distraction therapy and a tool to help decrease pain and anxiety.

3D Technology: Used in universities and hospitals, it is a learning tool for doctors, nurses, military medics, and first responders.

Augmented Reality (AR): The simplest way to describe AR is to understand the smartphone app Pokémon Go. It takes visual information, superimposes it on a real environment, and is akin to a hologram in space. AR is an ideal tool for patients who fear being in the fully immersive experience.

Design Thinking: Human-centered approach to tackling new problems and exploring new ideas with alternatives that haven't existed before (e.g., What do humans need? What makes life more enjoyable or easier? What makes technology practical and useful?).

Immersive Experience: Providing, involving, or characterized by deep absorption or immersion in something (such as an activity or a real or artificial environment).

Mixed Reality (MR): Encompasses the spectrum from Augmented Reality to Virtual Reality, blending the physical and digital worlds to produce new environments where physical and digital objects coexist and interact in real time.

Simulation: The act or process of stimulating, and the imitative representation of the functioning of one system or process by means of the functioning of another.

Telehealth: Telehealth is defined as the use of electronic information and telecommunication technologies to support long-distance clinical healthcare, patient and professional health-related education, public health, and health administration. Technologies include video conferencing, the Internet, store-and-forward imaging, streaming media, and terrestrial and wireless communications.

Virtual Reality (VR): VR is a completely immersed digital experience, providing a realistic simulation of a 3D environment that is experienced and controlled by movement of the body.

THOUGHT-PROVOKING QUESTIONS

1. Describe how immersive technologies increase patient satisfaction and improve outcomes.

2. In your estimation, when and how will your leadership bring VR/AR/MR into your clinical setting?

3. In the future, how might immersive technologies replace textbooks and lectures?

4. As a nursing educator, how likely is it that you would incorporate VR/AR/MR into your nursing programs? How will you accomplish this?

REFERENCES

Allcoat, D., & von Mühlenen, A. (2018). Learning in Virtual Reality: Effects on performance, emotion and engagement. *Research in Learning Technology, 26*, 2140. doi:10.25304/rlt.v26.2140

American Association of Colleges of Nursing. (2019). *The impact of education on nursing practice.* Retrieved from https://www.aacnnursing.org/News-Information/Fact-Sheets/Impact-of-Education

American Hospital Association. (2019, January 09). *For the 17th year in a row, nurses top Gallup's poll of most trusted profession.* Retrieved from https://www.aha.org/news/insights-and-analysis/2019-01-09-17th-year-row-nurses-top-gallups-poll-most-trusted-profession

American Nurses Association. (n.d.). *ANA strategic plan 2017–2020.* Retrieved from https://www.nursingworld.org/ana/about-ana/strategic-plan

Anderson, A., & Jiang, J. (2018, May 31). *Teens, social media & technology 2018.* Retrieved from https://www.pewinternet.org/2018/05/31/teens-social-media-technology-2018

Baker, M. (2017, September 18). *How VR is revolutionizing the way future doctors are learning about our bodies.* Retrieved from https://www.ucsf.edu/news/2017/09/408301/how-vr-revolutionizing-way-future-doctors-are-learning-about-our-bodies

Bellini, H., Chen, W., Sugiyama, M., Shin, M., Alam, S., & Takayama, D. (2016). Virtual & Augmented Reality: Understanding the race for the next computing platform. *Profiles in Innovation, 1.* Retrieved from https://www.goldmansachs.com/insights/pages/technology-driving-innovation-folder/virtual-and-augmented-reality/report.pdf

Bloomberg. (n.d.). *Company profile.* Retrieved from https://www.bloomberg.com/profile/company/715530Z:US?cic_redirect=2

Brightman, J. (2016, August 18). *VR/AR to reach $162 billion in worldwide revenues by 2020—IDC.* Retrieved from https://www.gamesindustry.biz/articles/2016-08-18-vr-ar-to-reach-usd162-billion-in-worldwide-revenues-by-2020-idc

Brown, T. (2009). *Transcript of "Designers—Think big!"* Retrieved from https://www.ted.com/talks/tim_brown_urges_designers_to_think_big/transcript#t-2799

Burbach, K. (2017, April 3). *UNMC celebrates naming, groundbreaking for iEXCEL home.* Retrieved from https://www.unmc.edu/news.cfm?match=20207

CAE Healthcare Videos. (2018, February 13). *CAE VimedixAR with Microsoft HoloLens Augmented Reality* [Video file]. Retrieved from https://youtu.be/1-ks5aJveCU

Canberra, U. O. (2017, October 19). *Nursing HoloLens at UC.* Retrieved from https://www.youtube.com/watch?v=_ORnPuJlAlU

Chakravarthy, B., Ter Haar, E., Bhat, S. S., McCoy, C. E., Denmark, T. K., & Lotfipour, S. (2011). Simulation in medical school education: Review for emergency medicine. *The Western Journal of Emergency Medicine, 12*(4), 461–466. doi:10.5811/westjem.2010.10.1909

Chan, E., Foster, S., Sambell, R., & Leong, P. (2018). Clinical efficacy of virtual reality for acute procedural pain management: A systematic review and meta-analysis. *PLoS One, 13*(7), e0200987. doi:10.1371/journal.pone.0200987

Chirico, A., Ferrise, F., Cordella, L., & Gaggioli, A. (2018). Designing awe in virtual reality: An experimental study. *Frontiers in Psychology, 8*, 2351. doi:10.3389/fpsyg.2017.02351

CISION-PRN Newswire. (2017, June 20). *Augmented Reality (AR) & VVrtual Reality (VR) in healthcare market is expected to reach USD 5.1 billion by 2025.* Retrieved from https://www.prnewswire.com/news-releases/augmented-reality-ar--virtual-reality-vr-in-healthcare-market-is-expected-to-reach-usd-51-billion-by-2025-300477030.html

Cook, A., Jones, R., Raghavan, A., & Saif, I. (2017, December 05). *Digital reality: The focus shifts from technology to opportunity*. Retrieved from https://www2.deloitte.com/insights/us/en/focus/tech-trends/2018/immersive-technologies-digital-reality.html

Cornish, A., & Gringlas, S. (2017, August 3). *Vermont Medical School says goodbye to lectures* [Audio file]. Retrieved from https://www.npr.org/sections/health-shots/2017/08/03/541411275/vermont-medical-school-says-goodbye-to-lectures

Craig, E., & Georgieva, M. (2017, August 30). *VR and AR: Driving a revolution in medical education & patient care*. Retrieved from https://er.educause.edu/blogs/2017/8/vr-and-ar-driving-a-revolution-in-medical-education-and-patient-care

Curtin, K. (2017, January 7). Mixed Reality will be most important tech of 2017. Retrieved from https://thenextweb.com/insider/2017/01/07/mixed-reality-will-be-most-important-tech-of-2017/

DeClercq, J., Bowen, M., Cotten, S. R., Hansen, A., Hebert, K., Nohel, J., Weber, K., Engler, K., & Marble, K. (2018). Improving care in the pediatric emergency department with virtual reality. *Iproceedings, 4*(2), e11796. doi:10.2196/11796

Deloitte. (2018). *2018 Global health care outlook: The evolution of smart healthcare* (pp. 1-31). Retrieved from https://www2.deloitte.com/content/dam/Deloitte/global/Documents/Life-Sciences-Health-Care/gx-lshc-hc-outlook-2018.pdf

Dimock, M., & Dimock, M. (2019, January 17). *Defining generations: Where Millennials end and Generation Z begins*. Retrieved from https://www.pewresearch.org/fact-tank/2019/01/17/where-millennials-end-and-generation-z-begins

Dudley, N., Ackerman, A., Brown, K., & Snow S.; American Academy of Pediatrics Committee on Pediatric Emergency Medicine; American College of Emergency Physicians Pediatric Emergency Medicine Committee; & Emergency Nurses Association Pediatric Committee. (2015). Patient-and family-centered care of children in the emergency department. *Pediatrics, 135*(1), e255–e272. doi:10.1542/peds.2014-3424

Dyer, E., Swartzlander, B. J., & Gugliucci, M. R. (2018). Using Virtual Reality in medical education to teach empathy. *Journal of the Medical Library Association, 106*(4), 498–500. doi:10.5195/JMLA.2018.518

Farber, O. N. (2018, August 14). *Medical students are skipping class in droves—And making lectures increasingly obsolete*. Retrieved from https://www.statnews.com/2018/08/14/medical-students-skipping-class

Fein, J. A., Zempsky, W. T., & Cravero, J. P.; Committee on Pediatric Emergency Medicine and Section on Anesthesiology and Pain Medicine. (2012). Relief of pain and anxiety in pediatric patients in emergency medical systems. *Pediatrics, 130*(5), e1391–e1405. doi:10.1542/peds.2012-2536

Fertleman, C., Aubugeau-Williams, P., Sher, C., Lim, A., Lumley, S., Delacroix, S., & Pan, X. (2018). A discussion of Virtual Reality as a new tool for training healthcare professionals. *Frontiers in Public Health, 6*, 44. doi:10.3389/fpubh.2018.00044

The Franklin Institute. (n.d.-a). *History of vVrtual Reality*. Retrieved from https://www.fi.edu/virtual-reality/history-of-virtual-reality

The Franklin Institute. (n.d.-b). *What's the difference between AR, VR, and MR?* Retrieved from https://www.fi.edu/difference-between-ar-vr-and-mr

Galea, S. (2019). *Well*. New York, NY: Oxford University Press.

Gaudiosi, J. (2015, October 16). *How Western University of Health Sciences is using Virtual Reality to teach students*. Retrieved from https://fortune.com/2015/10/16/western-university-is-using-virtual-reality-to-teach

Gershon, J., Zimand, E., Lemos, R., Olasov Rothbaum, B., & Hodges, L. (2003). Use of virtual reality as a distractor for painful procedures in a patient with pediatric cancer: A case study. *CyberPsychology & Behavior, 6*(6), 657–661. doi:10.1089/10949310 3322725450

Gershon, J., Zimand, E., Pickering, M., Rothbaum, B. O., & Hodges, L. (2004). A pilot and feasibility study of Virtual Reality as a distraction for children with cancer. *Journal of the American Academy of Child & Adolescent Psychiatry*, *43*(10), 1243–1249. doi:10.1097/01.chi.0000135621.23145.05

Global Industries Analysts, Inc. (2019). *Virtual (VR) in healthcare market trends*. Retrieved from https://www.strategyr.com/MarketResearch/Virtual_Reality_VR_In_Health care_Market_Trends.asp

Gold, J. I., & Mahrer, N. E. (2018, April). Is Virtual Reality ready for prime time in the medical space? A randomized control trial of pediatric Virtual Reality for acute procedural pain management. *Journal of Pediatric Psychology*, *43*(3), 266–275. doi:10.1093/jpepsy/jsx129

Guze, P. (2015). Using technology to meet the challenges of medical education. *Transactions of the American Clinical and Climatological Association*, *126*, 260–270. Retrieved from https://www.ncbi.nlm.nih.gov/pmc/articles/PMC4530721

Haluck, R. S. (2000). Computers and virtual reality for surgical education in the 21st century. *Archives of Surgery*, *135*(7), 786. doi:10.1001/archsurg.135.7.786

Heath, S. (2018, February 28). *How VR can boost individualized patient education, care experience*. Retrieved from https://patientengagementhit.com/news/how-vr-can-boost-individualized-patient-education-care-experience

Helsel, S. (1992). Virtual reality and education. *Educational Technology*, *32*(5), 38–42.

Heilbrunn, B. R., Wittern, R. E., Lee, J. B., Pham, P. K., Hamilton, A. H., & Nager, A. L. (2014). Reducing anxiety in the pediatric emergency department: A comparative trial. *Journal of Emergency Medicine*, *47*(6), 623–631. doi:10.1016/j.jemermed.2014.06.052

Jenson, C. E., & Forsyth, D. M. (2012). Virtual reality simulation: Using three-dimensional technology to teach nursing students. *CIN: Computers, Informatics, Nursing*, *30*(6),312–318. doi:10.1097/NXN.0b013e31824af6ae

Joynt, J., & Kimball, B. (2008, May 1). *Blowing open the bottleneck*. Retrieved from https://www.rwjf.org/content/dam/farm/reports/reports/2008/rwjf29362

Kent, C. (2019, May 20). *Cognitant Q&A: How Virtual Reality is reshaping patient information*. Retrieved from https://www.medicaldevice-network.com/digital-disruption/virtual-reality/vr-in-the-medical-field

Kilmon, C. A., Brown, L., Ghosh, S., & Mikitiuk, A. (2010). Immersive Virtual Reality simulations in nursing education. *Nursing Education Perspectives*, *31*, 314–317. Retrieved from https://journals.lww.com/neponline/Abstract/2010/09000/Immersive_Virtual_Reality_Simulations_in_Nursing.11.aspx

Klick Health. (2018, February 28). *Boston Children's Hospital & Klick Health Announce VR platform to offer pediatric patients customized 3D tours inside their bodies*. Retrieved from https://www.klick.com/health/announcements/boston-childrens-hospital-klick-health-announce-vr-platform-to-offer-pediatric-patients-customized-3d-tours-inside-their-bodies

Koller, D., & Goldman, R. (2012). Distraction techniques for children undergoing procedures: A critical review of pediatric research. *Journal of Pediatric Nursing*, *27*(6), 652–681. doi:10.1016/j.pedn.2011.08.001

Kyaw, B., Saxena, N., Posadzki, P., Vseteckova, J., Nikolaou, C., George, P., … Tudor Car, L. (2019). Virtual reality for health professions education: Systematic review and meta-analysis by the Digital Health Education Collaboration. *Journal of Medical Internet Research*, *21*(1), e12959. doi:10.2196/12959

Laerdal Medical AS. (2015, June 8). *vSim for nursing fundamentals online, virtual simulation* [Video file]. Retrieved from https://youtu.be/X2-qA433Uis

LaFreniere, H. (2017, March 2). *Foresight: TTUHSC peers into the future with Pearson*. Retrieved from https://dailydose.ttuhsc.edu/2017/march/LUB_Pearson_HoloLens.aspx

Lateef, F. (2010). Simulation-based learning: Just like the real thing. *Journal of Emergencies, Trauma, and Shock*, *3*(4), 348–352. doi:10.4103/0974-2700.70743

Lerwick, J. L. (2016). Minimizing pediatric healthcare-induced anxiety and trauma. *World Journal of Clinical Pediatrics*, *5*(2), 143–150. doi:10.5409/wjcp.v5.i2.143

Li, A., Montaño, Z., Chen, V. J., & Gold, J. I. (2011). Virtual reality and pain management: Current trends and future directions. *Pain Management*, *1*(2), 147–157. doi:10.2217/pmt.10.15

Li, S. (n.d.). *The role of simulation in nursing education: A regulatory perspective* [Slide set]. Retrieved from https://ncsbn.org/Suling2.pdf

Lippincott Nursing Education. (2017, March 14). *Nursing in a virtual world*. Retrieved from http://nursingeducation.lww.com/blog.entry.html/2017/03/15/nursing_in_a_virtual-UctW.html

Louie, A. K., Coverdale, J. H., Balon, R., Beresin, E. V., Brenner, A. M., Guerrero, A. P., & Roberts, L. W. (2018). Enhancing empathy: A role for Virtual Reality? *Academic Psychiatry*, *42*(6), 747–752. doi:10.1007/s40596-018-0995-2

Lowood, H. (n.d.). *Virtual Reality. Encyclopaedia Britannica*. Retrieved from https://www.britannica.com/technology/virtual-reality

MacLaren, J. E., Thompson, C., Weinberg, M., Fortier, M. A., Morrison, D. E., Perret, D., & Kain, Z. N. (2009). Prediction of preoperative anxiety in children: Who is most accurate? *Anesthesia and Analgesia*, *108*(6), 1777–1782. doi:10.1213/ane.0b013e31819e74de

Madathil, K. C., Frady, K., Hartley, R. S., Bertrand, J. W., Alfred, M., & Gramopadhye, A. K. (2017). An empirical study investigating the effectiveness of integrating virtual reality-based case studies into an online asynchronous learning environment. *Computers in Education Journal*, *8*(3), 1–10. Retrieved from https://www.asee.org/documents/papers-and-publications/papers/CoEd_Journal-2017/Jul-Sep/MADATHIL_EMPIRICAL.pdf

Mantovani, F., CasteInuovo, G., Gaggioli, A., & Riva, G. (2003). Virtual reality training for health-care professionals. *CyberPsychology & Behavior*, *6*(4), 389–395. doi:10.1089/109493103322278772

Maples-Keller, J. L., Bunnell, B. E., Kim, S.-J., & Rothbaum, B. O. (2017). The use of virtual reality technology in the treatment of anxiety and other psychiatric disorders. *Harvard Review of Psychiatry*, *25*(3), 103–113. doi:10.1097/HRP.0000000000000138

Maresky, H. S., Oikonomou, A., Ali, I., Ditkofsky, N., Pakkal, M., & Ballyk, B. (2019). Virtual Reality and cardiac anatomy: Exploring immersive three-dimensional cardiac imaging, a pilot study in undergraduate medical anatomy education. *Clinical Anatomy*, *32*(2), 238–243. doi:10.1002/ca.23292

Market Watch. (2019, April 30). *Mixed reality headset market is about to cross over 35 billion US dollars by 2024*. Retrieved from https://www.marketwatch.com/press-release/mixed-reality-headset-market-is-about-to-cross-over-35-billion-us-dollars-by-2024-2019-04-30

Murray, T. A. (2013). Innovations in nursing education: The state of the art. *Journal of Nursing Regulation*, *3*(4), 25–31.

Nager, A. L., Mahrer, N. E., & Gold, J. I. (2010). State trait anxiety in the emergency department: An analysis of anticipatory and life stressors. *Pediatric Emergency Care*, *26*(12), 897–901. doi:10.1097/PEC.0b013e3181fe90eb

National League for Nursing. (2015, April 20). *A vision for teaching with simulation: A living document from the National League for Nursing (NLN) Board of Governors*. Retrieved from http://www.nln.org/docs/default-source/about/nln-vision-series-(position-statements)/vision-statement-a-vision-for-teaching-with-simulation.pdf?sfvrsn=2

National League for Nursing. (n.d.-a). *Institute for Simulation and Technology*. Retrieved from http://www.nln.org/centers-for-nursing-education/nln-center-for-innovation-in-education-excellence/institute-for-simulation-and-technology

National League for Nursing. (n.d.-b). *Simulation*. Retrieved from http://www.nln.org/professional-development-programs/simulation

The NDP Group. (2018, September 11). *Over half of the 211.2 million video gamers in the U.S. play games across multiple platforms, according to NPD*. Retrieved from https://www.npd.com/wps/portal/npd/us/news/press-releases/2018/over-half-of-the-211-2-million-video-gamers-in-the-u-s--play-games-across-multiple-platforms--according-to-npd

Pappano, L. (2018, October 31). Training the next generation of doctors and nurses. *The New York Times*. Retrieved from https://www.nytimes.com/2018/10/31/education/learning/next-generation-of-caregivers.html

PennState University Libraries. (2019). *Virtual Reality services*. Retrieved from https://libraries.psu.edu/services/virtual-reality-services

Piromchai, P., Avery, A., Laopaiboon, M., Kennedy, G., & O'Leary, S. (2015). Virtual Reality training for improving the skills needed for performing surgery of the ear, nose or throat (Review). *Cochrane Database of Systematic Reviews*, (9), CD010198. doi:10.1002/14651858.CD010198.pub2

Reid Chassiakos, Y., Radesky, J., Christakis, D., Moreno, M. A., & Cross, C.; AAP Council on Communications and Media. (2016). Children and adolescents and digital media. *Pediatrics*, *138*(5), e20162593. doi:10.1542/peds.2016-2593

ReportBuyer. (2017, May). *Augmented Reality (AR) & vVrtual Reality (VR) in healthcare market analysis by component (hardware, software, and service), by technology (Augmented Reality, Virtual Reality), and segment forecasts, 2014–2025*. Retrieved from https://www.reportbuyer.com/product/4946492/augmented-reality-ar-and-virtual-reality-vr-in-healthcare-market-analysis-by-component-hardware-software-and-service-by-technology-augmented-reality-virtual-reality-and-segment-forecasts-2014-2025.html

Rodriguez, S., Caruso, T., & Tsui, B. (2017). Bedside entertainment and relaxation theater: Size and novelty does matter when using video distraction for perioperative pediatric anxiety. *Pediatric Anesthesia*, *27*(6), 668–669. doi:10.1111/pan.13133

Rodriguez, S., Munshey, F., & Caruso, T. J. (2018). Augmented Reality for intravenous access in an autistic child with difficult access. *Pediatric Anesthesia*, *28*(6), 569–570. doi:10.1111/pan.13395

Rogers, S. (2018, October 23). *Why millennials need VR*. Retrieved from https://www.forbes.com/sites/solrogers/2018/10/23/why-millennials-need-vr/#52c81a126260

San Diego State University. (2017, March). *School of Nursing: 21st century training comes to SDSU*. Retrieved from https://chhs.sdsu.edu/pulse-online/fallwinter-2017/son-6

Seymour, N. E., Gallagher, A. G., Roman, S. A., O'Brien, M. K., Bansal, V. K., Andersen, D. K., & Satava, R. M. (2002). Virtual Reality training improves operating room performance: Results of a randomized, double-blinded study. *Annals of Surgery*, *236*(4), 458–464. doi:10.1097/00000658-200210000-00008

Sharecare. (n.d.). *YOU*. Retrieved from https://www.sharecare.com/static/YOU

Stanford Children's Health. (2017). *The Stanford Virtual Heart—Revolutionizing education on congenital heart defects*. Retrieved from https://www.stanfordchildrens.org/en/innovation/virtual-reality/stanford-virtual-heart

Steele, E., Grimmer, K., Thomas, B., Mulley, B., Fulton, I., & Hoffman, H. (2003). Virtual Reality as a pediatric pain modulation technique: A case study. *CyberPsychology & Behavior*, *6*(6), 633–638. doi:10.1089/109493103322725405

Topol, E. (2015). *The patient will see you now*. New York, NY: Basic Books.

Trottier, E. D., Ali, S., Le May, S., & Gravel, J. (2015). Treating and reducing anxiety and pain in the paediatric emergency department: The TRAPPED survey. *Paediatrics & Child Health*, *20*(5), 239–244. doi:10.1093/pch/20.5.239

The University of Illinois College of Medicine. (2019). *Academic year 2019-20*. Retrieved from https://chicago.medicine.uic.edu/education/md-curriculum/curriculum-by-year/phase-1/m1-recommended-textbooks-and-materials

U.S. Department of Education. (n.d.). *Use of technology in teaching and learning.* Retrieved from https://www.ed.gov/oii-news/use-technology-teaching-and-learning

U.S. Department of Health and Human Services. (2019). *Telehealth programs.* Retrieved from https://www.hrsa.gov/rural-health/telehealth/index.html

Van Wagenen, J. (2017, July 19). *Medical schools get virtual with VR and AR trainings.* Retrieved from https://edtechmagazine.com/higher/article/2017/07/medical-schools-get-virtual-vr-and-ar-trainings-0

Weir, K. (2018, February). Virtual Reality expands its reach. *American Psychological Association, 49*(2), 52. Retrieved from https://www.apa.org/monitor/2018/02/virtual-reality

Western University of Health Sciences. (n.d.). *J and K Virtual Reality learning lab.* Retrieved from https://www.westernu.edu/virtualrealitylearningcenter

Wolitzky, K., Fivush, R., Zimand, E., Hodges, L., & Rothbaum, B. O. (2005). Effectiveness of Virtual Reality distraction during a painful medical procedure in pediatric oncology patients. *Psychology & Health, 20*(6), 817–824. doi:10.1080/14768320500143339

Wolters Kluwer: Lippincott Nursing Education. (2018, November 30). *VSim: A virtual simulation modality for today's nursing students.* Retrieved from https://www.youtube.com/watch?time_continue=9&v=5N8nWKn3IRE

Wolters Kluwer: Lippincott Nursing Education. (n.d.). *The future of technology in nursing education.* Retrieved from http://nursingeducation.lww.com/lp/nursing-education-technology-gif.html

Won, A. S., Bailey, J., Bailenson, J., Tataru, C., Yoon, I. A., & Golianu, B. (2017). Immersive Virtual Reality for pediatric pain. *Children (Basel), 4*(7), 52. doi:10.3390/children4070052

World Health Organization. (2019). *Priorities: Health for all.* Retrieved from https://www.who.int/dg/priorities/health-for-all/en

Yale School of Nursing. (n.d.). *Simulation and assessment lab.* Retrieved from https://nursing.yale.edu/academics/simulation-and-assessment-lab

Yuan, C., Rodriguez, S., Caruso, T., & Tsui, J. (2017). Provider-controlled Virtual Reality experience may adjust for cognitive load during vascular access in pediatric patients. *Canadian Journal of Anesthesia, 64*(12), 1275–1276. doi:10.1007/s12630-017-0962-5

Zhu, E., Hadadgar, A., Masiello, I., & Zary, N. (2014). Augmented Reality in healthcare education: An integrative review. *Peer J, 2*, e469. doi:10.7717/peerj.469

Zion Market Research. (2019, February 21). *Global augmented and virtual reality market will reach USD 814.7 billion by 2025.* Zion Market Research. Retrieved from https://www.globenewswire.com/news-release/2019/02/21/1739121/0/en/Global-Augmented-and-Virtual-Reality-Market-Will-Reach-USD-814-7-Billion-By-2025-Zion-Market-Research.html

ADDITIONAL RESOURCES

Capua, T., Kama, Z., & Rimon, A. (2018, March). The influence of an accredited pediatric emergency medicine program on the management of pediatric pain and anxiety. *Israel Journal of Health Policy Research, 7*(1), 17. doi:10.1186/s13584-018-0211-6

Chan, E., Hovenden, M., Ramage, E., Ling, N., Pham, J. H., Rahim, A., … Leong, P. (2019). Virtual Reality for pediatric needle procedural pain: Two randomized clinical trials. *The Journal of Pediatrics, 209*, 160–167.e4. doi:10.1016/j.jpeds.2019.02.034

Health Resources and Services. (2019, July 24). *Telehealth programs.* Retrieved from https://www.hrsa.gov/rural-health/telehealth/index.html

Hoffman, H. G., Patterson, D. R., Carrougher, G. J., & Sharar, S. R. (2001). Effectiveness of Virtual Reality-based pain control with multiple treatments. *The Clinical Journal of Pain, 17*(3), 229–235. doi:10.1097/00002508-200109000-00007

Parsons, T., Riva, G., Parsons, S., Mantovani, F., Newbutt, N., Lin, L., Venturini, E., & Hall, T. (2017). Virtual Reality in pediatric psychology. *Pediatrics, 140*(Suppl. 2), S86–S91. doi:10.1542/peds.2016-1758I

Pearson. (2016, October 26). *Pearson announces Mixed Reality pilots designed to solve real world learning challenges at colleges and universities.* Retrieved from https://www.pearson .com/us/about/news-events/news/2016/10/pearson-announces-mixed-reality-pilots -at-colleges-and-universities.html

The Pokémon Company. (2016). *Pokémon Go homepage.* Retrieved from https://www .pokemongo.com/en-us

Rodriguez, S., Tsui, J. H., Jiang, S. Y., & Caruso, T. J. (2017). Interactive video game built for mask induction in pediatric patients. *Canadian Journal of Anesthesia, 64*, 1073. doi:10.1007/s12630-017-0922-0

Stanford Chariot Program. (2017). *Our team.* Retrieved from https://chariot.stanford .edu/about

Yale School of Nursing. (2018, January 5). *Expansion of Yale School of Nursing's simulation lab.* Retrieved from https://nursing.yale.edu/news/expansion-yale-school-nursings-simulation-lab

5

The Internet of Things

THOMAS R. CLANCY

CONTENTS

INTRODUCTION

The phrase **the Internet of Things** (IoT) was first coined in 1985 as the integration of people, processes, and technology with connectable devices and sensors to enable remote monitoring, status, manipulation, and evaluation of trends of such devices. Since then, however, the IoT has become the enabler of a new paradigm that integrates machines, platforms, and the crowd through such technologies as **Artificial Intelligence (AI)**, robotics, and social media. This chapter will explore how the IoT interfaces with technology and humans to automate much of the work of nurses and create new knowledge through the "information value loop." The objective of this chapter is to discuss key factors driving the buildout of the IoT; how automation, AI, and robotics will transform nursing roles; and how to successfully plan for the future.

THE EVOLUTION OF AUTOMATION

At the turn of the 19th century nearly 50% of the workforce was employed in farming. Today, less than 2% of U.S. labor is employed in this area (U.S. Department of Agriculture Economic Research Service, 2019). In less than a century, the agricultural industry has completely transformed itself from a labor-intensive field to a fully automated one. Armed with self-driving combines embedded with AI, fields of crops that once took an entire community weeks to harvest can now be completed by a few individuals in a matter of days. Sitting in the cab of a $500,000 combine is not unlike sitting at the controls of a spaceship. Computer screens monitor multiple analytics such as the yield and moisture level of the various crops while complex algorithms control the height and speed of various harvesting and planting devices.

Farming took approximately 100 years to transition to full **automation**. Thus, there was sufficient time for farm laborers to change skillsets to new industries such as manufacturing. However, manufacturing has gone through a similar transition. For example, building cars at the turn of the century was a "job shop" process where one or two individuals built the entire car. With the advent of Henry Ford's assembly line process, the auto industry was able to mass produce cars by assigning individual tasks to laborers. Although this greatly expanded the manufacturing workforce, beginning in the 1970s assembly line workers began being replaced by robots. Today, up to 90% of the auto assembly line processes are now automated (Javalosa, 2017). It is important to note that unlike farming, this transition took approximately 50 years and resulted in insufficient time for many laborers to relearn skills needed in the new industries of today.

Blue-collar jobs, primarily in agriculture and various manufacturing industries, have thus far been impacted the most by advances in technology. However, with the dawn of the information age, service sectors are now in the crosshairs of a major transformation. For illustration, consider the travel industry. I recently took a business trip to Canada. From the time I checked in at the airport to picking up my baggage in Canada, I spoke to one person, and that was the Canadian customs agent. In other words, the entire air travel experience was fully automated. I checked in at a computer terminal to access my boarding pass, checked and weighed my bag via an automated machine, identified myself by a biometric scan of my eyes, boarded the plane with a bar code scanner, selected and watched a movie from the inboard Wi-Fi service, processed my passport in customs through an automated device that took my picture, spoke briefly with the customs agent, and then picked up my suitcase at the baggage claim from a conveyor belt.

These three examples highlight the evolution of change across multiple economic sectors caused by exponential advances in technology. It is estimated that in the next 10 years, 10 million jobs in existence today could be eliminated by machine automation (CBINSIGHTS, 2017). Jobs at one time thought to be insulated from automation are clearly in the crosshairs of change. Not only do these positions include non-healthcare professionals such as attorneys, paralegals, stockbrokers, and accountants but also healthcare professionals such as pharmacists, radiologists, and pathologists. Much of this change is driven by advances characterized by the use of **DANCE technologies,** which stands for: data, algorithms, networks, the cloud, and exponential growth (McAfee & Brynjolfsson, 2017). Combined, advances in DANCE technologies have facilitated the ongoing creation and growth of AI, while the IoT has increased access to it.

Given the relentless march of automation over the last century, what impact will AI, robotics, and the IoT have on healthcare, and specifically nursing, in the coming years? This chapter will discuss key factors driving the wave of automation soon to transform nursing, how AI and the IoT will enable this transformation, what nursing roles will be most vulnerable to change, and how to successfully plan for the future.

HOW INFORMATION GROWS

To understand the key factors behind the exponential advances in information technology it is important to start with defining the term "information." Contrary to what most individuals think, information theorists define "information" as the ordered arrangement of matter that represents something (Hildago, 2017). However, unlike the colloquial use of the term "information," meaning is not embodied in it. For example, the arrangement of atoms in a typical automobile represents information. However, although we know that the arrangement of atoms represents an automobile, it is the ordered structure of the atoms that is information. Information can also be represented by the arrangement of atoms in bits on a computer's hard disk. If one considers information as simply the ordered arrangement of matter, then it becomes easier to understand the challenges we face in processing it as it becomes more complex.

Information and complexity are closely associated. If we view the richness of information along a continuum, we find at one end complete randomness (e.g., the atoms bouncing around in a gas) and at the other end complete order (the arrangement of atoms in a crystal which simply repeat the same pattern over and over again). Neither example is very rich in information. The area between complete randomness and order is most rich in information, but it is also the area that is most complex and difficult to process. Take, for example, the arrangement of atoms that represents information in the multiple databases that make up an electronic health record (EHR) in a health system. Over time information begets more information and thus creates a driving force of increasing complexity. This is no more evident today than in the field of data science, which has emerged to manage, process, and analyze the massive amount of historical and new data being created daily.

If the sheer amount of new information today is contributing to complexity, then how does information grow? Since the dawn of man, our cognitive capacity has been dependent on the evolution of the human brain and its ability to process information. However, evolution is painstakingly slow, and even today's brightest individuals have limits to their cognitive capacity. Thus, as communities formed and ideas could be shared among its members, new ideas emerged and information grew. The buildout of roads coupled with new forms of transportation further extended access to more people and new knowledge. The recording of ideas through the written word and eventual invention of the printing press enabled the spread of knowledge at a pace never before experienced. The harnessing of steam and electricity during the industrial revolution created mass forms of transportation and communication. The invention of the computer and its ability to send and store information digitally further accelerated the growth of information. Today, the Intranet enables the sharing and processing of information at a rate of 66% new information per year (Varian & Lyman, 2003). We are now on the cusp of superintelligence as AI continues to be advanced and already exceeds human intelligence in certain areas.

The historical growth of information has been difficult to track over time. However, a surrogate measure of information growth is the global gross domestic product (GDP; Hildago, 2017). The GDP is defined as the total value of the goods and services produced by the people of a nation during a year. As information grows and innovation increases, the GDP represents the economic value of these new products and services. Historical GDP can accurately be estimated as far back as the 1500s where growth in GDP was flat. However, from the first industrial revolution in the early 1800s till today, GDP has grown at an exponential rate.

Linear Versus Exponential Growth in Information

Why is information growing at such a fast rate today? Much of this has to do with the transition of goods and services to a digital **platform**. For illustration, compare how an automobile is built to how a software program is developed. A software developer programs a new application by using digital code that, once created, can be copied accurately and instantly multiple times at virtually no cost. The software program can then be distributed to potential clients via the Internet for practically nothing. There is an exponential relationship between the resources required and the number of software applications copied. However, an automobile once built cannot be instantly copied and scaled up like a software program. There is a linear relationship between the number of cars built and the resources required. Each automobile produced requires the same amount of resources. However, once a software program is developed, it requires few resources to scale up. In other words, the information age is built on a digital platform where products and services can be scaled up accurately, instantly, and for free (McAfee & Brynjolfsson, 2017).

If it feels as though life is moving faster today than in the past, it likely is. The exponential growth in information is driving innovation and advances in new technology. We can see innovation at work through **Moore's law** which, over the last 40 years, has accurately predicted the rapid growth in computer chip processing power and storage capacity. According to the law, the number of transistors that can fit on a computer chip will double approximately every 18 months. This growth in transistors has literally doubled the processing power of computers every 2 years and been the driver of the exponential growth in information technology today (intel, n.d.).

The time between advances in succeeding new technologies is decreasing at a much faster rate than our ability to implement them. For example, the time between invention of the printing press, steam power, electricity, radio, telephone, and computer has decreased at an accelerating rate as the information processing tools of prior generations were used to make those of the next (The Singularity Is Near Webpage, 2019). Who would have thought prior to 2007 when the smartphone was first introduced that a device small enough to fit in your pocket could act as a phone, camera, global positioning system (GPS), calculator, video recorder, accelerometer, email, text and voice activation messaging service, Internet browser, flashlight, and many other functions. Each individual application integrated into a smartphone was at one time an invention unto itself. However, combining these individual applications to create yet a new device is also a form of innovation known as combinatorial innovation.

Combinatorial Innovation and Crossover

Combinatorial innovation was a key driver in the development of today's smartphone as many applications already existed. However, to successfully integrate those applications, developers needed to search for advances in technology across multiple fields. For example, GPS, initially developed in aerospace and naval research laboratories, has been integrated into multiple, disparate areas including the military, automotive industry, boating, and meteorology, to name a few (Committee on the Future of the Global Positioning System & Commission on Engineering and Technical Systems, 1995). Video cameras, initially invented by the gaming industry, are now integrated into security cameras, smartphones, the motion picture industry, and many other devices (Rewind Museum, n.d.; Charles Ginsberg, n.d.). What is important to note here is that advances in one field can "cross over" and lead to significant advances in other fields. Together combinatorial innovation and crossover have fueled growth in DANCE technologies and the emergence of a new technological paradigm that is characterized by **machines** that extend and enhance the individual human mind and body through AI; **platforms** that provide better access to products and services through the IoT; and **the crowd** that taps the wisdom of the human collective through social media (McAfee & Brynjolfsson, 2017). The next section of this chapter will focus on each of these key areas and how they will impact nursing care models in the future.

MACHINES, PLATFORMS, AND THE CROWD

Machines

In its simplest form, a machine is a mechanical structure that uses power to apply forces and control movement to perform an intended action. Machines also include computers and sensors that monitor performance and plan movement. As noted earlier, machines, through automation, have transformed virtually all sectors of the economy. But specifically, how has the emergence of DANCE technologies, the IoT, and AI impacted nursing? As discussed previously, nursing has been cited as "low risk" for automation. This is because the work of nurses is unpredictable, nonroutine, and requires caring and empathetic behavior, which is not something machines are good at. However, if you take a closer look, much of the work of nurses today is "semiautomated" and is actually following the same evolutionary path as in other fully automated industries.

THE FIRST WAVE OF AUTOMATION

The progression of automation within an industry generally follows a series of waves. The first wave begins by machines automating individual tasks that are routine, repetitive, predictable, and precise. If we look at common hospital nursing tasks, many meet these criteria. Table 5.1 lists four common nursing tasks and the degree to which they are routine, repetitive, predictable, and precise.

For example, medication administration in a hospital setting is semi-*routine* because it is performed on nearly all inpatients. It is *repetitive* because we administer medications daily on a schedule that is BID, TID, and so on. The outcomes are semi-*predictable* because most patients receive the medication's desired effect. And medication administration must be *precise* to avoid any adverse effects.

Although medication administration has not been fully automated, it has been semiautomated. Starting with medication dispensing by pharmacy, medications are placed in unit dose drawers by robots. The medication administration record (MAR) interfaces with the EHR and the seven rights (right person, medication, route, dosage, time, reason, and documentation) can, in part, be verified by bar code medication management systems. Note that one machine does not automate all of these nursing tasks; each function requires its own machine and software.

Table 5.1 The First Wave of Automation in Nursing: Routine, Repetitive, Predictable, and Precise

Activity	Routine	Repetitive	Predictable	Precise
Medication administration	Semi	Yes	Semi	Yes
Patient assessment	Yes	Yes	Semi	Yes
Scheduled vital signs	Yes	Yes	Yes	Yes
Clinical documentation	Yes	Yes	Yes	Yes

Routine: Core activities of acute care nursing
Repetitive: Activities that are done the same way and repeated
Predictable: Activities that are done every shift
Precise: Activities that need to be accurate (e.g., medication administration).

The same can be said for many other nursing tasks. Temperature, once obtained manually with a glass thermometer, is now automated by a device that can be swiped across the forehead or placed in the ear. Blood pressure, once taken with a manually inflated cuff and manometer, is now administered with a self-inflating cuff and a digital readout. Clinical documentation, once handwritten in paper charts, has now been replaced with automated text and typed notes in an EHR. There are even automated beds today that turn the patient from side to side. All of these individual nursing tasks, once performed manually, are now administered by machines in this first wave of automation.

THE SECOND WAVE OF AUTOMATION

The second wave of automation is driven by combinatorial innovation and cross-over from other industries. Existing technologies in healthcare are combined to create new technologies, many using technologies developed from non-healthcare industries. For example, there are now devices that can be placed on a patient's wrist that can be combined to continuously monitor blood pressure, pulse, and pulse oximetry (Caretaker Medical, 2018). Hands-free communication devices worn by a nurse can answer call lights, as well as facilitate communication between other nurses and outside telephone calls. Advances in cardiac ultrasound and electrocardiography allow both tests to be integrated into a small handheld device, eliminating the need for a stethoscope. Point of service handheld devices process lab tests at the bedside, eliminating the need to send specimens to a centralized lab. Smartphones gather data from biosensors and send them to the cloud via the Internet where they are processed for treatment of chronic diseases such as diabetes, asthma, and heart failure. These are just a few examples of the second wave of automation already sweeping healthcare.

Although automation is following a similar path in healthcare as in other sectors of the economy, nursing has not realized the gains in productivity seen in other industries. The use of EHRs, bar coded medication management, continuous physiologic monitoring, and other forms of automation have been shown to improve clinical outcomes and reduce medical errors but have not necessarily increased nurse productivity. In fact, staffing ratios have actually increased by 11.5% nationally since 2004 when California first legislated mandatory staffing ratios in hospitals (Conway, Konetzka, Jingsan, Volpp, & Sochalski, 2008; Staggs & He, 2013). That may bode well for job security in the near future, but if nursing cannot keep pace with the gains in productivity from automation seen in other industries, pressure to reduce expenses in other ways will continue to increase.

Nursing has some unique challenges when it comes to automation. In contrast to other industries, new technology tends to have little impact; in some cases, it increases labor costs in hospital nursing. For example, the rapid implementation of EHRs by hospitals to meet standards in the Accountable Care Act required hospitals to spend millions of dollars in equipment and implementation costs. However, studies have not consistently demonstrated improvements in nurse productivity, and in many cases have shown a decrease in it (Heath, 2016; Kutney-Lee, Sloane, Bowles, Burns, & Aiken, 2019; Poissant, Pereira, Tamblyn, & Kawasumi, 2005).

Hands-free communication devices such as Vocera® have been shown to decrease the amount of time nurses search for staff on the floor or answer patient call lights. Yet, there is no evidence to support changes in overall nurse staffing ratios. Digital thermometers take less time to measure a patient's temperature than a glass thermometer, but not enough to reduce staffing levels. One area that does appear to improve nurse productivity is video monitoring of fall risk patients that previously needed "sitters" stationed in their rooms. By allowing one technician to monitor several patients via a remote video monitoring system, the number of staff required to observe fall risk patients is significantly reduced.

For the immediate future, it would appear that the most we can hope for is the semi-automation of various nursing tasks as previously described. However, in the long run, nursing must find ways to further automate their work to achieve the same level of productivity gains seen in other industries and find solutions to an estimated shortfall of 1.09 million nurses by 2024 (American Association of Colleges of Nursing, 2019) due to nurse retirements and an aging population demographic. In the interim, short-term strategies to reduce the healthcare costs will concentrate on the third wave of automation by integrating advances in robotics, the IoT, and AI in nursing care.

THE THIRD WAVE OF AUTOMATION: AI, ROBOTICS, AND THE IoT

Artificial Intelligence

To understand the challenges of advancing to the third wave of automation, let's first start with a brief understanding of AI relating to IoT. Experts have turned to AI programs as an alternative because rather than simply computing an answer, they learn the structure of a dataset. AI methods, such as **machine learning**, are suitable for these types of problems because the accuracy of outcomes improves as more data are processed and algorithms are revised. Machine learning, **Big Data**, and better algorithms (Kelly, 2016) have significantly improved development of AI. In fact, computers already outperform humans in many areas today. Table 5.2 shows the year the reigning (human) world champion was beaten by computer for seven of the most popular games today.

The commercial transition of healthcare AI is being pioneered by a number of companies including IBM and Google. IBM's Watson supercomputer can assist

Table 5.2 Will Artificial Intelligence Eliminate Human Decision-Making? Where Computers Outperform Humans Today

Game	The Year a Computer Beat the Reigning Champion
Backgammon	1979
Chess	1997
Checkers	2002
Scrabble	2002
Bridge	2002
Jeopardy	2010
Go	2017

Source: Data from Bostrom, N. (2014). *Superintelligence: Paths, dangers, strategies.* Oxford, UK: Oxford University Press.

providers in diagnosing and making faster decisions through "cognitive computing," a platform that interacts through natural language processing to evaluate
disparate forms of data and learn from each interaction. Watson is currently being
used to optimize patient selection for clinical trials through intelligent matching.
For example, in oncology, these systems assist in the creation of individualized
treatment plans that enhance patient and experience. IBM Watson analyzes the
meaning and context of structured and unstructured data coming from a variety
of inputs including handwriting documents to match treatments most likely to
benefit patients (IBM, n.d.).

Google has also entered the healthcare market for AI with its DeepMind®,
a more open-ended, comparatively simpler platform to use than its competitors
because of its deep learning (DL) capabilities. Founded in London in 2010,
DeepMind utilizes data from the National Health Service to create unsupervised
learning algorithms for diagnosis of disease conditions and recommend treatment. Although both IBM Watson and Google DeepMind's goal is to augment
human intelligence through AI, their methods approach it differently (Alphabet,
Inc., n.d.).

Simply being able to process and analyze this sheer amount of data requires
a team of clinicians, data scientists, computer engineers, and others. To understand the challenges of today's data complexity, imagine a Rubik's cube as a
three-dimensional (3D) database spreadsheet. Your objective is to find a pattern
that represents the least number of steps needed to solve a Rubik's cube. If we
multiply six sides to every cube times 27, the total cubes in a Rubik's cube, there
are a total of 324 sides. If we consider each side a data element in the spreadsheet,
you have a 1 in 4.3×10^{19} chance of finding the solution by randomly searching
for it (Hildago, 2017)! Solving problems of this magnitude is not unusual in
healthcare, especially if the data have many different variables and are nonlinear.

Applications in Nursing   AI techniques, such as machine learning techniques, are
used in both nursing research and in practice today to analyze data and predict
outcomes and are intelligent systems that are increasingly being used in a number
of key areas in healthcare. Examples of machine learning applications include
classifying data into clinical dashboards and medical diagnosis and recommender
systems for treatment plans (medical, nursing), optimizing best practices (clinical
pathways), comparative effectiveness (drugs, technology, practice), prediction
(risk profiling: diabetes, stroke, MI, readmission, pressure ulcers, falls), personalized medicine (customized treatment plans based on genetic testing), healthcare
robots (locomotion and orientation to surroundings), sentiment analysis, classifying DNA sequences for diagnosis of disease conditions and natural language
processing, and voice activated communications for clinical documentation. For
example, Exhibit 5.1 represents the steps used to predict patients most at risk for
pain intolerance following surgery using decision trees.

In step 1, we begin by selecting a dataset and identifying concepts relevant
to our study with the help of domain experts and various statistical methods
such as factor analysis. Next, in step 2, we work with pain experts to review all
possible combinations of pain elements and remove factors we know do not
contribute to pain. Once we have identified the key data elements, we now allow,
in step 3, the computer to search for combinations of factors (called conjunctive

EXHIBIT 5.1
DECISION TREE: PREDICTIVE MODEL FOR POSTOPERATIVE PAIN

a. Step 1: Select concepts.
b. Step 2: Remove irrelevant factors.
c. Step 3: Search for positive conjunctive conjectures.
d. Step 4: Remove negative conjunctive conjectures.
e. Step 5: Build algorithmic rules around positive conjunctive conjectures.

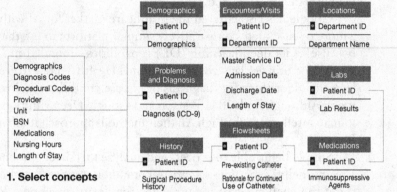

1. Select concepts

2. Remove irrelevant factors

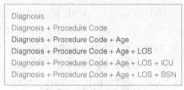

3. Search for positive conjunctive conjectures

4. Remove negative conjunctive conjectures

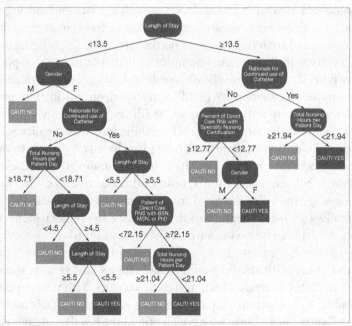

5. Build algorithmic rules around positive conjunctive conjectures

conjectures) that result in positive outcomes (pain intolerance). In step 4 we remove any negative conjectures (combinations that are not associated with pain). The remaining positive conjunctive conjectures can then be transformed into a hierarchy of rules (a decision tree) by the computer in step 5. Once trained on additional datasets, this model will predict which patients are at the highest risk for postsurgical pain intolerance.

AI: An Enabler or Eliminator of Jobs?   Given the recent advances in AI, what impact will this have on future healthcare workers? Jobs eliminated by AI take on a typical evolution. A good example is interpretation of radiology images. Currently, most of the AI applications within radiology are narrowly focused on achieving a specific task using DL, a subfield of AI, using layers of artificial neural networks. Areas of active DL focus within radiology include lesion detection, classification and diagnosis, segmentation, and quantification. The sensitivity and specificity of DL on accurately interpreting images varies considerably and depends on many factors. However, over time, as more data are processed through feedback mechanisms within DL neural networks, differences between machine and radiologist interpretations begin to narrow. Through this iterative process, it is possible, at some point in time in the future, that the majority of radiology images will be interpreted by pattern recognition software (McBee et al., 2018). In fact, this has already occurred in electrocardiogram interpretations, the majority of which are accurately interpreted by software, then over-read by a cardiologist (Exhibit 5.2).

EXHIBIT 5.2
HEALTHCARE VENTURE FUNDING

Artificial Intelligence/Machine Learning Funding Area

1 Research & Development Catalyst
2 Population Health Management
3 Clinical Workflow
4 Health Benefits Adm.
5 Diagnosis of Disease
6 Monitoring of Disease
7 Treatment of Disease
8 Clinical Decision Support and Precision Medicine
9 Nonclinical Workflow
10 Data Infrastructure & Interoperability
11 Prevention of Disease
12 Fitness & Wellness
13 Care Coordination
14 Consumer Health
15 Customer Acquisition & Relationship Management
16 Patient Adherence
17 On-Demand Healthcare Services
18 Marketplace
19 Medical Reference

Cumulative Venture Funding: Years 2011–2017

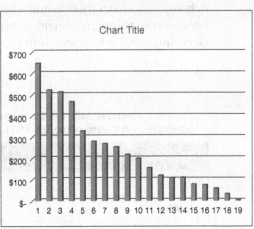

Rock Health: The AI/ML Use Case Investors Are Betting On in Healthcare. Accessed at rockhealth.com

Does this mean that AI embedded in today's EHRs will be making critical decisions regarding diagnosis and treatment of patients in lieu of medical providers? Many providers are concerned that they will be forced to comply with recommendations generated from AI software. However, a better question is how will AI support providers in making critical decisions? Today's AI performs best when it is programmed to solve specific types of problems such as those in games. This type of AI is called "narrow AI" and excels when tasks are easily broken down into sequential, smaller mathematical components. Most of today's AI is narrow AI. For example, the voice commands on smartphones are a form of narrow AI.

Strong AI represents the ability to apply intelligence to any problem rather than one specific problem. Also known as general intelligence, strong AI would equal or outperform human performance in any of the games previously mentioned. Strong AI software will likely continue to improve in the years to come, but when 100 top experts in AI were asked the question, "When will AI be equivalent to human general intelligence?" 50% indicated this would not be achieved until at least 2040 (Table 5.3; Bostrum, 2016).

Robotics

The second component to the third wave of automation is the emergence of **robotics** in healthcare. Except for a few areas such as pharmacy, lab, and supply chain management, the introduction of robots into the healthcare industry has been challenging. Because robots lack general intelligence, they are primarily limited to unifunctional tasks such as picking a medication from a shelf in pharmacy or delivering supplies to a floor. In terms of providing nursing care, robots tend to be extremely heavy and lack the finger dexterity needed for many patient care functions. And finally, the software used in robots lacks emotional intelligence, a key behavior required for healthcare providers (King, Lightman, Rangaswami, & Lark, 2016).

Robots also suffer a unique stigma not seen in other forms of technology. The idea of robots was, for decades, portrayed in books and movies before the technology had even been invented. In these settings, robots were often depicted as evil machines intent on conquering the world. Thus, the public's perception of robots interacting with humans has been unpopular from the start. Additionally, defining just what a robot is and what field they belong to is challenging. This is because robots integrate many fields including engineering, computer science, electronics, and informatics into their design (Jordan, 2016).

Table 5.3 When Will Machine-Level Intelligence Be Equivalent to Human Intelligence? A Survey of the Top 100 Experts in Artificial Intelligence

Year	Percent Chance (%)
2022	10
2040	50
2075	90

Source: Data from Bostrom, N. (2014). *Superintelligence: Paths, dangers, strategies.* Oxford, UK: Oxford University Press.

There is a perception that the computer software in robots must be located within the robot itself. However, if the expectation is that robots will need to have AI at a general intelligence level to perform multitasking, one would need the equivalent of a supercomputer in each robot. Clearly this is not practical, and robots today are more likely to have their intelligence controlled from the cloud in the IoT. To do so, multiple industries will have to collaborate to successfully integrate robotics into healthcare. This is particularly important as it applies to the implementation of robots by hospitals and clinics (Ford, 2016). In developing a robotics strategy for the future, one hospital department such as Information Systems or Engineering cannot be the sole "owner" of the technology. Ownership of robots must be shared among multiple departments.

Worldwide Growth in Robots   The simplest definition of a robot is a device that senses a signal, thinks about it, and then acts upon it. The key word is "think"; in this case, AI and cloud computing have contributed to the exponential growth of robotics (Jordan, 2016). For example, note the following facts regarding robots (King et al., 2016):

- Worldwide industrial robot growth has increased from 1 million robots in the year 2000 to 9 million in 2010, with 40% coming from Japan.
- Consumer robots are expected to grow from 6.6 million in 2015 to an estimated 31 million by 2020.
- By the year 2025, it is estimated that there will be 1.5 billion combined industrial and commercial robots worldwide.
- Industrial robot growth is estimated to outnumber the human population by 2030 and replace 50% to 70% of the jobs in the future.

Nursing and Robots   The integration of robots into hospitals has been slow, but what if you had no choice but to automate the work of nurses? This happens to be the case in Japan where the percentage of the population over age 65 years is near 25% and expected to grow to 40% by 2050 (King et al., 2016). The U.S. demographic is also heading toward a similar age distribution in the years to come and, like Japan, may be forced to automate certain aspects of nursing care. Similar to the theme we saw previously, individual nursing tasks in Japan are in the process of being automated. There are exoskeleton robots that assist patients walking up stairs, telepresence robots that can enter a room and connect a specialist in a different hospital to an inpatient, robots that pick up and deliver supplies to a nursing unit, companion robots to keep the elderly company in senior homes, and even robots that can wash the patient's hair. The Japanese government is funding two thirds of any research for new technology that can reduce the number of nurses needed in the future (King et al., 2016). So, it is quite possible that we will start to see combinatorial innovation and crossover in robotics much sooner than we thought.

Duke University School of Nursing has taken a different approach with Rethink Robotics' Baxter® robot, a lightweight humanoid manufacturing robot that can easily be trained to perform a variety of repetitive tasks (Li, Moran, Dong, Shaw, & Hauser, 2017). In contrast to industrial robots, which require complex and expensive programming when changing tasks, Baxter can be trained simply by moving its arms through the required motions. If a facility uses multiple robots, one Baxter can be trained and then the software can be copied to the others (or scaled up) simply by plugging into a USB device. The history of computing shows that once a standard operating system together with inexpensive and easy-to-use programming tools becomes available, an explosion of application software is likely to follow (King et al., 2016). For example, Duke University's Engineering School in partnership with the Duke University School of Nursing was able to demonstrate that Rethink Robotics' Baxter robot could successfully carry out 23 simulated nursing tasks.

The next wave of robots will likely integrate the technology of telepresence, voice activation, cloud computing, the IoT, sensors, and AI and emotional intelligence to create humanoid-like robots through combinatorial innovation and crossover. However, will this be advanced enough to achieve the same improvements in productivity seen in other industries? To do so, health systems will need to create a robotics strategy that progressively creates value for the organization as the technology evolves. This might begin by utilizing robots to perform simple unifunctional tasks such as delivering materials to the hospital floors, telepresence mobile units for specialists, and companion robots for the elderly. As robot technology advances though, early adopters will be the first to experiment, pilot, and develop best practices that result in improved productivity and clinical outcomes. This will be a distinct advantage given the accelerating learning curve other economic sectors have experienced with the introduction of new technology.

Platforms

The second leg of the new paradigm in healthcare is platforms. "A platform is a group of technologies that are used as a base upon which other applications, processes, or technologies are developed" (Technopedia, n.d.). The IoT is one example of a platform and was formally defined in 1985 as the integration of people, processes, and technology with connectable devices and sensors to enable remote monitoring, status, manipulation, and evaluation of trends of such devices (The Internet of Things, Classic VOX website, 2017). Specifically, the IoT connects and sends digital messages between machines (computers, medical devices, and other) and between humans and machines (voice, audio, text, images, and so forth). With an estimated 50 billion devices embedded with sensors worldwide by 2020, the IoT will play a major role in enabling the new paradigm of machines, platforms, and the crowd (McCabe, 2016).

The IoT has emerged as DANCE technologies, facilitated by Moore's law, have resulted in smaller, faster, and less expensive devices, sensors, and networks. For example, the price of sensors has consistently fallen over the past several years and these price declines are expected to continue into the future. Over the last two decades, the speed and power of microprocessors has doubled every 18 months. The average number of sensors on a smartphone has increased from three (accelerometer, proximity, and ambient light) in 2007 to at least 10 (including advanced sensors such as fingerprint- and gesture-based sensors) today (Mahto & Varia, 2019).

GROWTH OF THE IoT PLATFORM

Advancements in networks and power consumption have also followed Moore's law. In the last 30 years, data rates have increased from 2 kbps to 1 Gbps, facilitating faster transfer of large data files. Communication messages have transitioned from analog to digital signals. The transit prices of the Internet have decreased due to the global increase in submarine cabling, the rising use of wavelength division multiplexing by Internet service providers (ISPs), the transition to higher-capacity bandwidth connections, and increased completion among service providers. The power capacity of batteries for mobile devices and sensors has not kept pace with the increased demands for processing data. To alleviate some of these problems, the introduction of low-energy Bluetooth has reduced power consumption energy by 50% when compared with Bluetooth classic (Mahto & Varia, 2019).

Better network standards between devices have also significantly enabled the IoT. For example, IPv4, the current system used to identify different devices, is limited by the total number of ID numbers it can provide. To solve this problem, companies are transitioning devices to the new ID system, IPv6, and by 2018, 50% of all fixed and mobile device connections are expected to be IPv6-based (Mahto & Varia, 2019).

Interoperability between devices has been challenging as today's existing technology standards serve specific solutions and stakeholder requirements. However, standards development by both vendors and professional associations such as the Institute of Electrical and Electronics Engineers and European Telecommunications Standards Institute are starting to develop unified standards related to the messaging, collection, handling, ownership, use, and sale of the data. There is also a growing need for regulation across the IoT as it relates to protected health information. For example, the U.S. Health Insurance Portability and Accountability Act (HIPAA, 1996) governs the protection of medical information collected by providers, hospitals, and insurance companies. However, the act does not extend to information collected through personal wearable devices (Mahto & Varia, 2019).

The IoT and Information Value Loop   Although many barriers still exist today, the IoT in combination with advances in AI will likely revolutionize healthcare delivery in the future. That is because the IoT connects machines, platforms, and the crowd, and enables the creation of value from new information. For example, we know that if a patient is administered a medication, it is likely to have the desired effect. This *current information* came from years of clinical trials and day-to-day medical practice. However, if a biosensor is embedded in the same medication, *new information* is created. For instance, we can now determine if the patient is taking the medication at a time that optimizes its therapeutic effect (especially important for certain kinds of oncology medications). This new information can then be transferred wirelessly via the Internet to the cloud where it is analyzed. Using various AI methods, recommendations can be made to *augment our current intelligence* and support clinical decision-making. Finally, this new information can be used to *augment the patient's behavior* through technology. For example, a smartphone application could be used to alert the patient when to take the medication to achieve its optimal therapeutic effect. This information is then revised through machine learning systems in the cloud to improve its accuracy each time the medication is taken. The iterative process of creating data, transferring it via networks to the cloud, creating new information from the data, transmitting it to healthcare providers to augment their intelligence, and finally providing it to the patient through technology to augment their behavior has been described as the "information value loop" (Mahto & Varia, 2019; Raylor & Cotteleer, 2019).

The IoT is driving the information value loop through advancements in DANCE technologies and Moore's law. These innovations will expand existing nursing roles as the IoT allows access to care and treatment of disease conditions once limited to only hospitals and clinics. For example, biosensors embedded in clothing can measure body temperature and electrocardiographic signals in heart failure patients. Sensors embedded in smartphones can detect sleep apnea in patients that could lead to heart attack or stroke. Digital scales can measure whether a patient is in fluid overload through impedance measurements. Smartphone sensors can measure the level of pollution in the air to alert patients with asthma. Motion detectors in patients' homes can detect an increase in trips to the bathroom at night and alert providers of a possible urinary tract infection. Smart pills can monitor a patient's adherence to his or her medication schedule. Biosensors can evaluate blood glucose levels and regulate continuous insulin pumps in diabetics. The list goes on and on.

As combinatorial innovation and technological crossover from different industries progresses, groups of sensors will be deployed for specific disease conditions. For example, chronic asthmatics may one day be able to prevent an acute attack by alerts from air quality sensors in their smartphones. This may prompt the individual to connect a device to his or her smartphone that allows the individual to conduct spirometry tests, oximetry, and other physiologic measurements. These data are then sent to the cloud, analyzed, and a recommendation is sent back to the individual to use his or her inhaler to actually *prevent* the asthma attack. Therefore, understanding how medical devices can be optimized within the IoT to create information value loops will be an important skillset for nurses in the future. Such nurses will act as healthcare information brokers by utilizing the IoT to reduce admissions and readmissions to hospitals by extending safe care into the home.

Venture Capital, the IoT, and Emerging Technologies   With the accelerating speed at which DANCE technologies advance today, it is difficult to predict which ones will be most successful in healthcare. One method is to monitor which healthcare areas are receiving the most **venture capital funding**. For example, Table 5.4 presents, in descending order, the key healthcare areas funded by venture capital companies for AI commercial applications in 2018 (Zweig & Tran, 2019).

After research and development, key areas of funding for AI are population health, clinical workflow, health benefits administration, diagnosis, treatment and monitoring of disease, clinical decision support, and precision medicine. All of these areas would benefit from AI applications for better management of chronic disease populations, best practices for clinical workflow in EHRs, predictive models for diagnosis of disease conditions, recommender systems based on evidence-based guidelines, and customized treatment plans using precision medicine.

The IoT will play a major role in facilitating access to AI through a number of emerging technologies, including IoT. Exhibit 5.3 lists some of the new technologies receiving major funding from venture capital companies that could impact nursing. These technologies include Augmented Reality (AR), Virtual Reality (VR), and conversational AI.

Table 5.4 Augmented, Virtual, and Artificial Intelligence

Technology	Activity	Market Leaders
Augmented Reality, Mixed Reality	Smart glasses that display: EHR vital sign, orders, notes, reports	Magic Leap, Microsoft HoloLens
Virtual Reality	Educational and training, surgery	Oculus Rift, Magic Leap, Microsoft
Conversational AI: Chatbots and personal assistants	Task list reminders and new order alerts. Advice and information on best practices. Hands-free execution of orders. Orientation of new staff.	Amazon Alexa, Microsoft Cortana, Google Smartphone Assistant, Apple Siri, IBM Watson

EHR, electronic health record.

EXHIBIT 5.3

AI SYSTEMS: AN ELIMINATOR OR ENABLER OF HEALTHCARE JOBS?

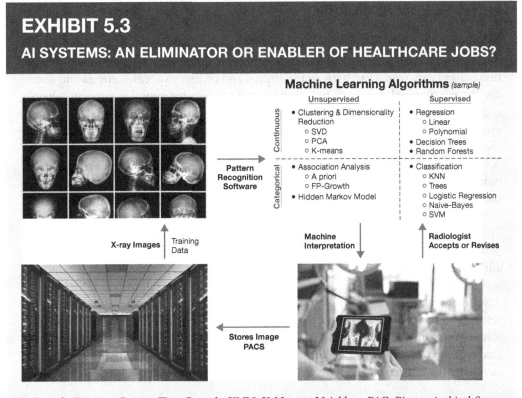

FP Growth, Frequent Pattern Tree Growth; KNN, K-Nearest Neighbor; PAC, Picture Archival System; PCA, Principle Component Analysis; SVD, Singular Value Decomposition; SVM, Support Vector Machine.

Augmented, Virtual Reality, Personal Assistants, and IoT   VR uses software to simulate 3D images, sounds, and sensations to isolate and surround you while AR overlays views of the physical world with fabricated images that engage users (Geyer, 2016). Conversational AI, also known as **chatbots**, act as personal assistants to answer questions and make recommendations to users. AR devices have the potential to create dashboards for nurses that can be viewed on computer screens or heads up display glasses (HUDs). Through the IoT, a HUD could connect to the hospital's cloud servers to provide pattern recognition software and identify a patient as a nurse enters his or her room. An IoT wireless connection to the hospital EHR could then transmit an AR dashboard of relevant information to the nurse's HUD glasses and a personal assistant could make care recommendations. Additional information from the EHR could be accessed and documented by the nurse through voice activated sensors in the HUDs. Individually, all of these devices and applications exist today. However, through crossover and combinatorial innovation, these applications will someday be fully integrated through the IoT and complete the information value loop.

CASE STUDY 5.1

INSPIREN'S iN: USING THE INTERNET OF THINGS AND AI TO INCREASE SAFETY AND QUALITY, AND ENHANCE PATIENT-CENTERED CARE

Development of IoT-based technology married with AI is becoming a way to enhance the quality of care provided to patients in many healthcare organizations. One way that patient care teams can harness intelligent and connective technologies and leverage their functionality is with IoT devices and ecosystems aimed to prevent adverse events, errors, and near misses in the delivery of care. In the United States, medical errors are the third leading cause of death with more than 250,000 deaths per year (Schwab, 2018), with the contributing factor of patient neglect to those events (Reader & Gillespie, 2013). Today, emerging technologies can lend their power to reduce these numbers and negate patient neglect to improve safety and clinical practice through the remote monitoring of people and objects in the patient care environment.

Determining the unknown patterns of routines, workflows, and environmental events in hospital rooms that change critical care routines are essential in reducing patient harm. With the mission to better understand patient care routines, mitigate adverse events, and improve patient outcomes, a team of practicing clinicians, nurses, and technologists at Inspiren, a New York-based start-up established in 2016, have developed an AI-powered IoT device to fight patient neglect and assist patient care teams in improving the quality of patient care delivery. Inspiren's nurses and technologists' invention of a hybrid sensing, wall-mounted, cognitive patient care assistant, iN, analyzes the real-time physical and digital patient environment to eradicate the harm caused by human error (P. Coyne, personal written communication, June 3, 2019). The

(continued)

CASE STUDY 5.1 (*continued*)

successful deployment of iN at two major hospitals in New York (The Medical Futurist [TMF], 2018) marks a movement toward improving patient safety and outcomes.

The start-up is leading technological innovation by assembling and directing an international team of engineers, data scientists, software developers, designers, and researchers from institutions such as NASA, MIT, and Columbia University (Coyne, 2019) for product development. Active collaboration of clinicians and technologists created iN's system to fully integrate with electronic health records (EHRs) and leverage computer vision, deep learning, low-energy Bluetooth, and natural body-movement recognition capabilities for a complete end-to-end patient care solution encompassing hardware, software, smart mobile health technology, and advanced analytics to monitor threats to patient safety.

The wall-mounted device detects staff presence and assesses environmental safety risks while simultaneously collecting and aggregating data from other medical devices such as ECGs, vital sign monitors, ventilators, and point-of-care (POC) devices. In addition, iN detects temperature, noise, and brightness, among other environmental factors in patient rooms (TMF, 2018). iN aggregates and intelligently delivers these data in real time via the care teams' mobile platform and utilizes nudge theory and gamification to distribute immediate feedback when staff display desirable action (Coyne, 2019). Also, iN's data analytics engine uses AI to create predictive algorithms to prevent future patient injuries and preventable errors and calculates patient workload to enhance staffing (TMF, 2018), as well as the care team's productivity and efficiencies. The layering of multiple technologies enables data capture to become fully automated, and the burden of documentation is lifted from patient care teams, allowing them to spend more high-value time with patients at the bedside (Coyne, 2019).

The iN device communicates with patient care teams using LED color signals. For example, a blue light indicates staff presence or shows the device is in use, a purple light shows the care team is present in a patient room, a green light indicates a safe care environment, and an orange light alerts staff when the patient requires attention based on the connected remote monitoring devices (Houghton, 2018). The real-time data transmit to an AI-enabled hospital-wide dashboard that reports care routine metrics including total in-room patient visits, missed rounding times, number of call bells activated, and number of bedside reports completed (Schwab, 2018). Nurses can leverage this cloud-based device to use actionable decision-making from the IoT data to improve patient care and also gather information for the broader healthcare organizations that can use them to reduce costs associated with adverse events, staffing level inefficiencies, and waste.

Inspiren's novel technology embodies the philosophy that patient care staff should be spending as much time with their patients as possible and also utilizing the technology to impart actionable data capture to ensure that nurses are rewarded and recognized for their delivery of safe, high-quality patient-centered care (Coyne, 2019). To date, a pilot with an academic medical center validated iN's IoT and AI technology capabilities, and Columbia University School of Nursing is publishing research demonstrating the system's impact on patient safety, patient satisfaction, nurse satisfaction, and compliance with hospital protocols (Coyne, 2019).

To conclude, a platform is a group of technologies that are used as a base upon which other applications, processes, or technologies are developed. The IoT is an evolving platform that integrates people, processes, and technology with connectable devices and sensors to enable remote monitoring, status, manipulation, and evaluation of trends of such devices. The IoT enables the "information value loop" by creating, transmitting, gathering, and analyzing data to create augmented intelligence for nurses and drive augmented behavior in patients. The integration of machines and platforms is democratizing healthcare services once available only in hospitals and clinics and dramatically changing nurses' roles. Nurses in the future will be evaluated, in part, by their ability to optimize the integration of machines and the IoT to improve patient care.

The Crowd

SOCIAL MEDIA, NEW ECONOMIES, AND THE IoT

The emergence of **social media** is the final component driving the new paradigm of machines, platforms, and the crowd. Social media is defined as electronic communication, such as through websites and applications, that enable users to create and share content or to participate in social networking. The integration of the IoT with social media websites offers health systems a valuable tool for social data aggregation on patients, providers, and business and industry (see Exhibit 5.3 and Figure 5.1).

It is also changing how care is provided and evaluated. For instance, the following is a list of healthcare areas that have been impacted by social media:

- **Patients and Families**—Inquiries regarding a patient's condition in a hospital were primarily through phone calls to nursing units, but online messaging services such as Caringbridge® now provide regular patient updates to those registered with the website.
- **Support Groups**—Traditionally, support groups used to meet face to face and were often mediated on-site by healthcare personnel. However, multiple support groups for many different disease conditions are now self-organized and meet continuously online. The website Healthfinders .gov sponsored by the Office of Disease Prevention and Health Promotion offers a search browser of hundreds of online support groups (https:// healthfinder.gov/FindServices/SearchContext.aspx?topic=833&Branch =6&show=1).
- **Public Health Departments**—The spread of disease or epidemics has historically been delayed because of the difficulties tracking it in real time. But by using pattern recognition software to track specific browser search terms and social media sites, researchers can predict where the disease may be spreading to next.
- **Human Resources**—Social media can be used to reference potential job applicants. By screening applicant behavior on social media sites such as Facebook, Twitter, and others, human resource departments may be able to reject applicants who demonstrate undesirable behavior online.

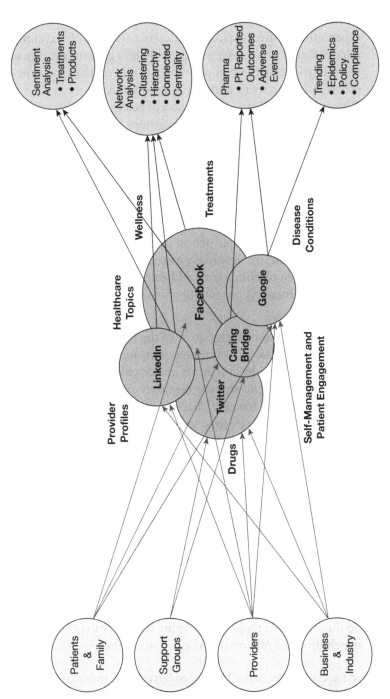

Figure 5.1 Healthcare social media data analysis.

- **Pharma**—Historically, medication errors, adverse events, and others were difficult to monitor outside of the hospital. However, pharmaceutical companies can now monitor outpatients through online discussion groups and monitor any medication events or reactions caused by their drugs.
- **Business and Industry**—Business and industry now regularly crowdsource experts from a diverse pool of industries to help solve complex problems once assigned to research groups in their organizations. These events are often introduced as a competition and rely on the crossover effect from different industries to find a unique solution.
- **Patient Satisfaction**—Satisfaction of healthcare services used to be conducted through surveys and focus groups but now are provided through source comments on Facebook, Twitter, LinkedIn, and other social media sites using sentiment analysis methods.
- **Referral Tracking**—The historical process used to define health system markets used to be manual and cumbersome. However, network analysis tools allow health systems to track referral patterns through a variety of social media sites.

These are just a small sample of how integration of the IoT with social media sites will impact healthcare. It is likely too early to tell whether social media will result in the creation or elimination of healthcare jobs in the future. However, they clearly are augmenting our intelligence through the information value loop.

THE SHARING ECONOMY

The IoT has also enabled development of the **sharing economy**, an ecosystem comprised of individuals, communities, companies, organizations, and associations where human and physical assets are shared among members. Healthcare has been slow to adopt the sharing economy model when compared to other sectors of the economy. However, that is changing as powerful apps are tapping the unused capacity of nurse's time to fill gaps in staffing.

Sharing economies are characterized by the following attributes (Penn & Wihbey, 2016):

- They use information technology, typically available via web-based platforms, such as mobile "apps" on Internet-enabled devices, to facilitate peer-to-peer transactions.
- They rely on user-based rating systems for quality control, ensuring a level of trust between consumers and service providers who have not previously met.
- They offer the workers who provide services via digital matching platform flexibility in deciding their typical working hours.
- To the extent that tools and assets are necessary to provide a service, digital matching firms rely on the workers using their own resources.

Sharing economies have facilitated growth in independent or "freelance" workers, which are expected to make up the majority of the U.S. workforce by 2027 (Upwork, 2017). By digitally matching individuals through apps, unused human capacity can be utilized with reduced effort by "intermediaries" such as a staffing office in a hospital or a commercial staffing agency. This lowers the transaction cost of the service and benefits both the customer and the provider.

The On-Demand Economy

One aspect of today's sharing economy is **on-demand economy** services such as Uber® and Lyft®. Through powerful apps, these services match the unused capacity of a driver and his car with individuals needing a ride. By developing very user-friendly software, Uber allows peer-to-peer (P2P) digital matching of driver to passenger with virtually no intermediary. Research has shown that by lowering transaction costs, overall Uber fares are lower and customer satisfaction is equivalent or higher when compared to traditional taxi services (Telles, 2016). The same can be said for many other on-demand services such as lodging (Airbnb®), entertainment (Netflix®), and retail (eBay®), to name but a few.

A number of challenges confront healthcare organizations as they attempt to implement similar on-demand services. These include existing business platforms and healthcare regulatory pressures. For example, commercial nurse staffing agencies have acted as intermediaries for providing on-demand staffing services to healthcare organizations for many years. However, because of regulatory requirements, hospital staffing agencies must gather and maintain a significant amount of ongoing documentation related to the nurses they employ. This documentation includes demographic information, background checks, references, competency evaluations, and many other forms of information.

Nurse staffing agencies also maintain a centralized pool of operators that frequently act as intermediaries between healthcare organization staffing offices and agency nurses to field questions and confirm assignments. Finally, healthcare organizations and staffing agencies are on different staffing software platforms and must manually input nurses into their respective schedules. Thus, the combination of meeting Centers for Medicare and Medicaid Services and The Joint Commission requirements, the need for agency schedulers, and disparate software systems leads to high overhead costs for staffing agencies. These costs are then passed onto healthcare organizations through the agency nurses.

In contrast, the only requirements related to Uber drivers are (Telles, 2016):

- You must be 21 years of age or older (23 depending on your city).
- The intended driver is required to be on the insurance for the vehicle used.
- You must pass a background check.
- A minimum of 3 years driving experience is mandatory.
- You are required to have a clean driving record.

Uber evaluates the competency and passenger satisfaction by simply having the passenger rate the driver (and vehicle) using a five-star rating system integrated into the Uber app.

Although on-demand nurse staffing has significant challenges as compared to ride sharing services, some early adopter health systems are beginning to utilize the model. A number of commercial apps are now available that wirelessly transmit "blasts" of open shifts to nurses in a convenient and easy-to-use format (Demand Workforce®, 2019). Some health systems, like Uber, are experimenting with developing an online rating system to evaluate nurses' performance on the unit. Other organizations have implemented a pay the next day process or "Quick Pay" to incentivize nurses to pick up shifts. Although each of these programs stands alone today, crossover and combinatorial innovation will likely integrate all of these functions into one app in the future.

CONCLUSION

Multiple sectors of the economy have improved productivity and eliminated blue-collar jobs by automating processes through new technology. The transition to automation is accelerating farming (100 years), manufacturing (40 years), and services (20 years). The shift to automation will continue at its relentless pace because, in the digital world, bytes are fast, perfect, instant, and free. White-collar jobs (including nursing) are now in the crosshairs of automation as DANCE technologies transition knowledge work to a new paradigm. The global economy is transitioning to a new paradigm that has been enabled through the integration of machines, platforms, and the crowd. Machine automation in healthcare has lagged as compared to other industries but is catching up quickly. Advances, driven by DANCE technologies, have automated many areas in hospitals, specifically in laboratory, radiology, and pharmacy departments. Nursing tasks, however, remain primarily semiautomated but are advancing through combinatorial innovation and AI. Given the success of automation in other fields, coupled with an anticipated shortage of nurses in the future, increased pressure will be placed on providers to manage populations through precision health and improve productivity through automation. The Intranet has exploited the wisdom of crowds by providing a platform to freely share information among its participants. By doing so, patients, providers, business, and industry can directly access group sentiment regarding health services, clinical treatments, patient satisfaction, and other by eliminating intermediaries. It has also created a digital marketplace where technology companies fill consumer demand via immediate access to goods and services (aka the on-demand economy). One example in nursing is in staffing where software apps can tap the unused capacity of nurses (the crowd) in other hospitals to fill surges in patient census quickly (Uberization of staffing). Combined, direct access to the "crowd" unleashes innovative ideas and lowers cost through disintermediation.

GLOSSARY

Artificial Intelligence: The aptitude exhibited by smart machines broken down into perceiving, thinking, planning, learning, and the ability to manipulate objects.

Automation: The technique of making equipment, a process, or a system operate automatically.

Big Data: Datasets, whose size is beyond the ability of typical database software tools to capture, store, manage, and analyze.

Chatbots: A computer program designed to replicate conversation with human users.

DANCE Technologies: An abbreviation that stands for data, algorithms, networks, the cloud, and exponential growth.

Machine Learning: Smart machines that learn over time automatically through experience, emphasize predictions, evaluate results via prediction performance, and serve to highlight algorithm performance and robustness of outcomes.

Moore's Law: How overall processing power for computers will grow exponentially over time.

On-Demand Economy: Lucrative activity created by technology companies that fulfill consumer demand through immediate provisioning of goods and services.

Platforms: Computer architecture and machinery using specific operating systems.

Robotics: The science and technology behind the design, manufacturing, and application of robots, programmable mechanical devices that can perform tasks and interact with their environment, without the aid of human interaction.

Sharing Economy: An ecosystem comprised of individuals, communities, companies, organizations, and associations where human and physical assets are shared among members.

Social Media: Electronic communication creates online communities to share information, ideas, personal messages, and other content.

The Crowd: The network that taps the wisdom of the human collective through social media.

The Internet of Things: The integration of people, processes, and technology with connectable devices and sensors to enable remote monitoring, status, manipulation, and evaluation of trends of such devices.

Venture Capital Funding: A method of funding a new or growing business from firms specializing in building high-risk financial portfolios in exchange for equity in the company, which are generally in rapid growth industries such as technology.

THOUGHT-PROVOKING QUESTIONS

1. If technology eventually eliminates the need for nurses to directly assess patients' clinical measurements (blood pressure, pulse, temperature, heart sounds, and so forth), should these skills still be taught in nursing schools?

2. If a robot can accurately mimic empathy and caring to support a patient, does it matter if those do not come from a human?

3. If a machine can more accurately diagnose and treat an illness than a human, what role will healthcare providers play in the future?

4. How can health systems today prepare for the changing roles of nurses impacted by automation?

REFERENCES

Alphabet, Inc. (n.d.). Alphabet, Inc accessed at the Wikipedia website on December 2, 2019, at https://en.wikipedia.org/wiki/Alphabet_Inc

American Association of Colleges of Nursing. (2019). *Nursing shortage fact sheet.* Retrieved from https://www.aacnnursing.org/News-Information/Fact-Sheets/Nursing-Shortage

Bostrom, N. (2014). *Superintelligence: Paths, dangers, strategies.* Oxford, UK. Oxford University Press.

Caretaker Medical. (2018). *CE certification approval for Caretaker®4 continuous non-invasive blood pressure (CNIBP) & wireless vital signs monitor.* Retrieved from http://www.caretakermedical.net/ce-certification-approval-for-caretaker-4-continuous-non-invasive-blood-pressure-cnibp-wireless-vital-signs-monitor

CBINSIGHTS. (2017). *AI will put 10 million jobs at risk.* Retrieved from https://www.cbinsights.com/research/jobs-automation-artificial-intelligence-risk

Charles Ginsberg. (n.d.). Obituary for Charles Ginsberg, *New York Times.* Accessed on December 2, 2019, at https://www.nytimes.com/1992/04/17/us/charles-p-ginsburg-71-leader-in-developing-video-recording.html

Committee on the Future of the Global Positioning System and Commission on Engineering and Technical Systems. (1995). *The global positioning system: A shared national asset: Recommendations for technical improvements and enhancements* (p. 16). Washington, DC: National Academies Press. Retrieved from https://www.nap.edu/read/4920/chapter/11

Conway, P. H., Konetzka, T. R., Jingsan, Z., Volpp, K. G., & Sochalski, J. (2008). Nurse staffing ratios: Trends and policy implications for hospitalists and the safety net. *Society of Hospital Medicine, 3*, 193–199. doi:10.1002/jhm.314

Demand Workforce. (2019). Retrieved from http://www.demand-workforce.com

Ford, M. (2016). *Rise of the robots: Technology and the threat of a jobless future*. Boston, MA: Basic Books.

Geyer, S. (2016). *What will augmented and virtual reality technology do for healthcare?* Retrieved from http://www.healthcareitnews.com/news/what-will-augmented-and-virtual-reality-technology-do-healthcare

Health Insurance Portability and Accountability Act of 1996, Public Law 104-191 (1996).

Heath, S. (2016). *92% of nurses dissatisfied with EHR technology, Health IT.* Retrieved from https://ehrintelligence.com/news/92-of-nurses-dissatisfied-with-ehr-technology-health-it

Hildago, C. (2017). *Why information grows: The evolution of order, from atoms to economies*. New York, NY: Basic Books.

Houghton, L. (2018). *Inspiren reduces patient vulnerability with new technology*. Retrieved from https://www.lsnglobal.com/news/article/22576/inspiren-reduces-patient-vulnerability-with-new-technology

IBM. (n.d.). *How to get started with cognitive technology*. Retrieved from https://www.ibm.com/watson/advantage-reports/getting-started-cognitive-technology.html

intel. (n.d.). *Fueling innovation we love and depend on*. Retrieved from https://www.intel.com/content/www/us/en/silicon-innovations/moores-law-technology.html

The Internet of Things, Classic VOX website. (2017). *Introduction to Internet of Things-IoT*. Retrieved from https://www.organworks.com/index.php/articles/306-introduction-to-internet-of-things-iot

Javalosa, J. (2017). *Production soared after this factory replaced 90% of its employees with robots*. Retrieved from https://www.weforum.org/agenda/2017/02/after-replacing-90-of-employees-with-robots-this-companys-productivity-soared

Jordan, J. M. (2016). *Robots*. Boston, MA: MIT Press.

King, B., Lightman, A., Rangaswami, J. P., & Lark, A. (2016). *Augmented: Life in the smart lane*. Singapore, Singapore: Marshall Cavendish International.

Kutney-Lee, A., Sloane, D. M., Bowles, K. H., Burns, L. R., & Aiken, L. H. (2019). Electronic health record adoption and nurse reports of usability and quality of care: The role of work environment. *Applied Clinical Informatics, 10*(01), 129–139. doi:10.1055/s-0039-1678551

Li, Z., Moran, P., Dong, C., Shaw, R., & Hauser, K. (2017). Development of a tele-nursing mobile manipulator for remote care-giving in quarantine areas. *2017 IEEE International Conference on Robotics and Automation (ICRA)*, Singapore. doi:10.1109/ICRA.2017.7989411

Mahto, M., & Varia, H. (2019). *The Internet of Things: A technical primer*. Retrieved from https://www2.deloitte.com/insights/us/en/focus/internet-of-things/technical-primer.html?icid=dcom_promo_featured|us;en

McAfee, A., & Brynjolfsson, E. (2017). *Machine, platform, crowd: Harnessing our digital future*. New York, NY: W. W. Norton.

McBee, M. P., Awan, O. A., Colucci, A. T., Ghobadi, C. W., Kadom, N., Kansagra, A. P., … Auffermann, W. F. (2018). Deep learning in radiology. *Academic Radiology, 25*(11), 1472–1480. doi:10.1016/j.acra.2018.02.018

McCabe, B. (2016). *Quick history of the Internet of Things*. Retrieved from https://www
.semiwiki.com/forum/content/5559-quick-history-internet-things.html

Penn, J., & Wihbey, J. (2016). *Uber, Airbnb and consequences of the sharing economy: Research
roundup*. Retrieved from https://journalistsresource.org/studies/economics/business/
airbnb-lyft-uber-bike-share-sharing-economy-research-roundup

Poissant, L., Pereira, J., Tamblyn, R., & Kawasumi, Y. (2005). The impact of electronic
health records on time efficiency of physicians and nurses: A systematic review.
Journal of the American Medical Informatics Association, 12(5), 505–516. doi:10.1197/
jamia.M1700

Raylor, M., & Cotteleer, M. (2019). *The more things change: Value creation, value capture,
and the Internet of Things*. Retrieved from https://www2.deloitte.com/insights/us/
en/deloitte-review/issue-17/value-creation-value-capture-internet-of-things.html

Reader, T. W., & Gillespie, A. (2013). Patient neglect in healthcare institutions: A
systematic review and conceptual model. *BMC Health Services Research, 13*, 156.
doi:10.1186/1472-6963-13-156

Rewind Museum. (n.d.). *Umatic. The 1st VCR & 1st ever portable VCR*. Retrieved from
http://www.rewindmuseum.com/umatic.htm

Schwab, K. (2018, July 19). *Patient neglect kills. This AI could help stop it*. Retrieved from
https://www.fastcompany.com/90204532/patient-neglect-kills-this-ai-could-stop-it

Staggs, V. S., & He, J. (2013). Recent trends in hospital nurse staffing in the United States.
Journal of Nursing Administration, 43(7–8), 388–393. doi: 10.1097/NNA.0b013e31829d620c

Technopedia. (n.d.). *Platform*. Retrieved from https://www.techopedia.com/definition/3411/
platform

Telles, R. (2016). *Digital matching firms: A new definition in the "Sharing Economy"
space. U.S. Department of Commerce Economics and Statistics Administration Office of the Chief Economist*. Retrieved from https://intuittaxandfinancialcenter
.com/wp-content/uploads/2017/02/digital-matching-firms-new-definition-sharing
-economy-space.pdf

The Medical Futurist. (2018). *Inspiren fights patient neglect with A.I.* Retrieved from
https://mailchi.mp/medicalfuturist/inspiren-fights-patient-neglect-with-ai-medical
-futurist-newsletter-special

The Singularity Is Near Webpage. (2019). *Countdown to singularity*. Retrieved from http://
www.singularity.com/charts/page17.html

Upwork Website. (2017). *Freelancers predicted to become the U.S. workforce majority within
a decade, with nearly 50% of millennial workers already freelancing, annual "Freelancing
in America" study finds*. Retrieved from https://www.upwork.com/press/2017/10/17/
freelancing-in-america-2017

U.S. Department of Agriculture Economic Research Service. (2019). *Farm economy: Farm
labor*. Retrieved from https://www.ers.usda.gov/topics/farm-economy/farm-labor

Varian, H., & Lyman, P. (2003). *How information grows*. Retrieved from http://kk.org/
thetechnium/the-speed-of-in

Zweig, M., & Tran, D. (n.d.). *The AI/ML use case investors are betting on in healthcare*. Retrieved from https://rockhealth.com/reports/the-ai-ml-use-cases-investors-are-betting
-on-in-healthcare

ADDITIONAL RESOURCE

U.S. Bureau of Labor Statistics. (n.d.). *Employment by major industry sector*. Retrieved from
https://www.bls.gov/emp/tables/employment-by-major-industry-sector.htm

6

Precision Health and Genomics

KATHLEEN A. McCORMICK

CHAPTER OBJECTIVES

- Describe the difference between Precision Medicine and Precision Health and Nursing's contributions to Precision Health.
- Understand the pharmacogenomics guidelines and the implications for nursing practice across the continuum of care.
- Discuss the four ways that nurses can participate in Precision Health.
- Identify the linkage between genomics information and informatics and understand the components of nursing informatics.
- Summarize some of the future technologies and challenges as nurses support genomics.

CONTENTS

(continued)

CONTENTS (*continued*)

INTRODUCTION

The force in this century that is bringing us into the Fourth Industrial Revolution requiring Artificial Intelligence (AI), machine learning (ML), robotics, clouds, and Big Data is the human genome. The human genome has only been known since 2001, but it is now expanding in the areas of prevention, diagnosis, and treatment throughout the continuum of care from preconception to end of life. The volume of data is increasing and necessitating secure clouds for storage and AI to span the multiple databases containing genetic reference data, imaging data, and clinical electronic health records (EHRs). This chapter describes the necessary definitions to understand Precision Health, genomics, pharmacogenomics, and some common examples of genomics throughout the continuum of care with a focus on symptom management and pharmacogenomics. The informatics needs for bioinformatics and Precision Health will be discussed. Specific nursing recommendations are provided. Barriers and challenges include nursing education, ethics, culture in society, and reimbursement.

PRECISION HEALTH

Congress signed legislation into law entitled the 21st Century Cures Act (2016). The law supports the Department of Health and Human Services (DHHS) to advance Precision Medicine by furthering research in disease prevention, diagnosis, and treatment, as well as implementing greater data sharing of genetic/genomic information. A part of this mandate to the National Institutes of Health (NIH) is the All of Us Research Program that has begun to collect the genetics/genomics

Table 6.1 Contributors to Health and Their Percentages

Lifestyle and behaviors—smoking, obesity, nutrition, blood pressure, alcohol, and drug use	40%
Genomics—related to human biology	30%
Environment—including social networking and living location	20%
Access to healthcare	10%

Source: Data from Schroeder, S. A. (2007). We can do better—Improving the health of the American people. *New England Journal of Medicine, 357*, 1221–1228. doi:10.1056/NEJMsa073350

of 1 million or more Americans from diverse ethnic backgrounds. Because the person's health may be modulated by different lifestyles—the environment that he or she lives in—new technologies are being developed to track these persons at home and everywhere the person goes. Some of these devices include tracking wearables and home devices that measure personal health and correlate it to overall health outcomes. **Precision Health** necessitates integrating these new devices with health records. Precision Health aims not only to cure diseases but also to prevent disease before it becomes manifest and improve symptom management during diagnosis and treatment in acute and chronic illness (NIH All of Us Research Program, n.d.).

Dr. Steven Schroeder described contributors to health. This was published in his Shattuck Lecture that was based on the contributions of Health versus Medicine from the World Health Organization (Schroeder, 2007). The contributors to health and their percentages that Schroeder described are listed in Table 6.1; they are lifestyle and behaviors (40%) such as smoking, obesity, stress, nutrition, blood pressure, alcohol, and drug use; genomics (30%) related to human biology; environment (20%) including social networking and living location; and access to healthcare (10%) through hospitals and community healthcare including outpatient care.

BASICS OF GENE STRUCTURES: LIKE READING BOOK

In the book *Genome* by Matt Ridley (1999), the author has the reader imagine that reading the gene is like reading a book. The updated definitions are from the National Human Genome Research Institute's (NHGRI's) Talking Glossary (https://www.genome.gov/genetics-glossary).

The 23 chromosome pairs make up 23 chapters of the book of life. Each set of 23 chromosomes contains approximately 3.1 billion base pairs of DNA sequence.

The chapters include stories called genes. The gene is the basic physical unit of inheritance. Genes are passed from parents to offspring and contain the information needed to specify traits. Humans have approximately 20,000 to 23,000 genes arranged on their chromosomes. The *BRCA2* gene alone contains 83,736 base pairs.

The stories include paragraphs called exons that are a part of the gene that codes for amino acids, which become proteins. Introns are the parts of the gene sequence that are not expressed in the protein because they come in between—or interfere with—the exons.

Each paragraph is made up of words called codons. A codon is a trinucleotide sequence of DNA or RNA that corresponds to a specific amino acid. The cell reads the sequence of the gene in groups of three bases. There are 64 different codons: 61 specify amino acids, while the remaining 3 are used as stop signals.

Each word is written in letters called bases. The essential letters are ACTG, which stand for *A*denine, *C*ytosine, *T*hymine, and *G*uanine. The genetic code describes the relationship between the sequence of DNA bases (A, C, T, and G) in a gene and the corresponding protein sequence that it encodes.

Assuming 400 pages are in a book, the human genome would occupy at least 262,000 pages or 175 large books. We are only 1% different in our genetic makeup from each other, which means only about 500 pages would be unique to us.

In the book *Genomic Medicine*, Guttmacher, Collins, and Drazen in 2004 took the next step to basically understand and describe the role of proteins (Guttmacher, Collins, & Drazen, 2004). Proteins are an essential class of molecules found in all living cells. A protein is composed of one or more long chains of amino acids, the sequence of which corresponds to the DNA sequence of the gene that encodes it. Proteins play a variety of roles in the cell, including structural (cytoskeleton), mechanical (muscle), biochemical (enzymes), and cell signaling (hormones). There are about 22,000 protein-coding genes in humans. This chapter will focus on the enzymes used to metabolize drugs in the area of pharmacogenomics.

CURRENT-DAY UNDERSTANDING OF THE BASICS

Recent discoveries have led to a more dynamic understanding of the science behind genomics so that the processes of the cells; molecules such as RNA and protein; and additional metabolites can be measured (Regan, Engler, Coleman, Daack-Hirsch, & Calzone, 2018). These discoveries are uncovering the underpinnings of health and disease, as well as the potentially precise treatment. The regulation of proteins (proteomics) is influenced by how genes transcribe into RNA in cells and tissue. Measuring the protein levels and their interactions can reveal more molecular mechanisms of disease. Also, the measurement of metabolic processes (metabolomics) demonstrates the influences on the gene to the environment, including food, bacteria in the body, and other microorganisms (microbiomes) in the body that contribute to health and disease.

In acquiring disease (especially cancer), two basic types of mutations have been identified: (a) somatic mutations that occur because of a mutation and (b) germline mutations that are present in the parent's sperm or egg and can be inherited. Germline mutations result in families with the disease. The older the father, the higher the mutation rate increases. Every time a mother gives birth to a child, he or she incurs 100 to 200 new mutations.

BASIC DEFINITIONS

There are four definitions in this chapter we need to understand that come from the *Scope and Standards of Nursing Practice* (American Nurses Association [ANA], 2015) and the area of OMICS.

Genetics—The study of individual genes and their impact on relatively rare single-gene disorders (NHGRI, n.d.-b)

Genomics—The study of all of the genes in the human genome together, including their interactions with each other, their environment, and other psychosocial and cultural factors (NHGRI, n.d.-b).

OMICS—The study of gen*omics*, prote*omics*, transcript*omics*, and metabol*omics*.

Pharmacogenomics—A branch of pharmacology concerned with using DNA and amino acid sequence data to inform drug development and testing. An important application of pharmacogenomics is correlating individual genetic variation with drug responses (NHGRI, n.d.-c).

TWO NURSING STANDARDS RELEVANT TO PRECISION HEALTH

The ANA added the concept of genetics and genomics to the *Nursing Informatics: Scope and Standards of Practice*, Second Edition (ANA, 2015). These standards inform nurses that they must be able to incorporate genetic and genomic technologies and informatics into practice and demonstrate in practice the importance of tailoring genetic and genomic information and services to clients based on their culture, religion, knowledge level, literacy, and preferred language. These principles are relevant to (a) Documentation of a RAPID risk assessment and (b) family history and ethnicity.

The second standard is the ANA *Principles for Nursing Documentation: Guidance for Registered Nurses*—nursing documentation standards indicate nurses must assess if the medication is appropriate to the patient's diagnosis, if the dose is appropriate, what the reaction to the medication is, and whether there are adverse reactions to the medication (ANA, 2010).

These principles of documentation are of relevance to (c) medication administration and documentation and (d) evaluation of medication adverse reactions. Professional practice license mandates on medication administration ordered by a physician or nurse practitioners (NPs) suggest (or require) implementing pharmacogenomics into nursing practice.

NURSING'S HISTORY OF ENGAGEMENT IN GENETICS/GENOMICS THROUGHOUT THE CONTINUUM OF CARE

Box 6.1 lists the categories of nursing's engagement in genetics and genomics throughout the continuum of care.

Box 6.1 Contributors and Percentage of Total Health

1. Preconception and prenatal healthcare
2. Newborn screening
3. Understanding of health, risks, and susceptibility for disease, therapy decisions, potentials to develop new therapeutic treatments, and responses to diagnoses and treatments
4. Screening and diagnosis
5. Prognosis and therapeutic decisions
6. Monitoring disease progression and symptom management

Preconception and Prenatal Healthcare

There are articles and recent book chapters by McCormick and Calzone (2016) discussing nursing's history of engagement in genetics/genomics throughout the continuum of care. The 3.9 million nurses in the United States and most nurses worldwide are familiar most with the use of genetics in the *preconception and prenatal healthcare continuum*. Preconception tests involve identifying the status of prospective parents for genetic variants associated with conditions such as sickle cell disease, Down syndrome, Edwards syndrome, multiple myeloma, cystic fibrosis, and Tay–Sachs disease (McCormick & Calzone, 2016). In the whole continuum of genetics/genomics testing, prenatal testing accounts for the highest percentage of genetic testing (Phillips, Deverka, & Hooker, 2018).

Newborn Screening

Nurses should be aware of genetic testing during *newborn screening*. After an infant is born, but before leaving the hospital or birth center, the infant's heel is pricked. A few drops of blood from the heel are then tested for certain genetic disorders such as hearing, congenital heart disease, endocrine, and metabolic disorders. As of 2019, there are 34 newborn screenings listed on the Recommended Uniform Screening Panel (RUSP) put forward by the Health Resources and Services Administration (HRSA, 2019). These conditions include phenylketonuria (PKU), cystic fibrosis, sickle cell disease, critical congenital heart disease, hearing loss, and others. According to the Centers for Disease Control and Prevention (CDC, 2018), about 3% to 6% of babies have a serious birth defect detected from newborn screening. Gene panels focus on a few dozen to a few hundred genes. Another observational assessment that can be determined by genomics is for glucose-6-phosphate dehydrogenase (G6PD) in infants, which suggests infant jaundice. A G6PD deficiency results in neonatal hyperbilirubinemia. If left untreated, this can result in kernicterus, cerebral palsy, and death (Kaplan & Hammerman, 2008).

Understanding Health Risks and Susceptibility for Disease and Therapy Response

The genetics and genomics in the healthcare continuum also provide us with an understanding of health, risks, susceptibility for disease, therapy decisions, potentials to develop new therapeutic treatments, and responses to diagnoses and treatments. Disease risks and susceptibility are done to determine inherited cancer syndromes such as breast, ovarian, and prostate syndromes associated with mutations in the *BRCA1* and *BRCA2* genes. Determining the hereditary nature of cancer accounts for the second highest percentage of spending on genetic/genomic tests (Phillips et al., 2018). Another example of risk and susceptibility that nurses are familiar with involves hypercholesterolemia associated with mutations in genes.

Screening and Diagnosis

The advances in *screening and diagnosis* genomics have accelerated in laboratories throughout the United States and globally because of direct-to-consumer (DTC) testing and approval by the U.S. Food and Drug Administration (FDA) of a popular DTC panel in the United States. Today, about 75,000 genetic tests are available from laboratories in every state in the United States (Phillips et al., 2018). It has been reported that there are about 10 new genetic tests available per week. The acceleration in genetic screening and diagnosis can also be attributed to the decline in the cost of sequencing the genome. The cost has decreased from $100 million in 2001 to less than $1,000 in 2014 (NHGRI, 2019b). The growth of DTC testing is also enhanced by telephone advertising of multiple tests, mobile apps, telemedicine capabilities, online portals for communicating between consumers and providers, YouTube, and Skype, with geneticists and counselors throughout the world interpreting health, pharmacogenomics, and metabolic and exercise genomics.

In April 2017, the FDA authorized 23andMe to market DTC tests that provide information on an individual's genetic predisposition to Parkinson's disease and late-onset Alzheimer's disease. In March 2018, the FDA approved DTC screening tests that authorized the personal genome service genetic health risk (GHR) for *BRACA1/BRACA2*, which is a breast cancer gene mutation of people of Ashkenazi (Eastern European) Jewish descent (FDA, 2017a). Other DTC companies provide the test kits to analyze DNA collected from a self-collected saliva sample. DTC genomics companies, like 23andMe, Ancestry.com, and Helix.com, are growing fast because of the number of consumers participating in their genetic testing.

FoundationOne CDx is the first FDA-approved broad companion diagnostic (CDx) that is clinically and analytically validated for solid tumors (FDA, 2017b). The test is designed to provide physicians with clinically actionable information—both to consider appropriate therapies for patients and understand results with evidence of resistance—based on the individual genomic profile of each patient's cancer. The first FDA-approved diagnostic testing with Medicare coverage includes all solid tumors, including non–small cell lung cancer (NSCLC), colorectal, breast, ovarian, and melanoma (FDA, 2017b).

Prognosis and Therapeutic Decisions

The next area of the continuum is in *prognosis and therapeutic decisions*. Prognosis and therapeutic decisions involve the area where so much growth and so many discoveries are occurring. There are currently 10,703 human variations of genomes of clinical significance in a database called ClinVar (National Center for Biotechnology Information [NCBI], U.S. National Library of Medicine [NLM], n.d.-a) and 2.4 million studies reported in another database at NIH called db-GaP (NCBI, NLM, n.d.-b). An example is prognosis and therapeutic decisions in the management of patients with acute myeloid leukemia (AML) that rely on genetic tests that inform diagnosis and prognosis, predict response to therapy, and measure minimal residual disease.

There are also about 2,000 rare and common diseases that can be identified by genetic testing. Also, there are 2,938 articles categorized in the National Library of Medicine (NLM) at the NIH, characterizing clinical effectiveness, disease, and drug studies (Genetic and Rare Diseases Information Center, 2018). To date, the use of genomic testing is occurring in the majority of hospitals (Shrestha, 2018). Genomic testing has been mostly in large academic and specialty care hospitals but is expanding to many community hospitals and to the Department of Defense (DoD).

Making headlines during the American Society of Clinical Oncology (ASCO) meeting in June 2018 were two trials using genomics in cancer. One project called TAILORx that was funded by the NIH was the most extensive breast cancer study ever (NIH, 2018). The findings demonstrated that 70% of 10,200 women with hormone receptor-positive, HER2-negative, ancillary node-negative early-stage breast cancer and a mid-range score on a 21-tumor gene expression test (using Oncotype DX® Breast Recurrence Score) did not need chemotherapy after surgery. The corollary was that 30% of the women did need chemotherapy. This study demonstrates that women can be spared the chemotherapy side effects of nausea, hair loss, and early menopause, and patients can save millions of dollars in chemotherapy costs. The genomic tests cost about $4,500, and the chemotherapies range from $40,000 to 80,000 for the extent of treatment.

In another privately funded study called ImPACT taking place at MD Anderson Cancer Center in Texas, the research team has found that in a personalized medicine trial, where they matched the tumor type with prospective treatments, prolonged survival in patients occurred with many tumor types (MD Anderson Cancer Center, 2018). They found that a patient's 3-year survival was 15% compared to 7% where tumor and treatment were not matched. After 3 years, 11% of over 1,307 patients were alive (MD Anderson Cancer Center, 2018).

Monitoring Disease Progression and Symptom Management

The final area of the continuum most relevant to nursing is *monitoring disease progression and symptom management*. Understanding the recurrence of disease, malignancy, and spread of diseases to additional organs has progressed using genetic, genomic, and protein databases. In the past, the genetics and genomics were being developed for cancer disease stages, as well as progression and symptom management. Today, the research is progressing for many health conditions, but specifically for cardiovascular disease, stroke, arthritis, amyotrophic lateral sclerosis (ALS), HIV, multiple sclerosis (MS), type 1 and 2 diabetes, Parkinson's disease, and depressive disorders.

The Role of Nursing in Precision Health

Clinical nursing has not embraced Precision Health as much as nursing research. The special role that nursing has carved out in Precision Medicine is through Precision Health, which develops and applies new knowledge in biology combined with behaviors, including genomics biomarkers, to improve patients' symptoms.

Nursing science is being conducted at the National Institute of Nursing Research (NINR) at the NIH. This Precision Health research focuses on nurses' ability to better understand the symptoms of many acute and chronic illnesses, such as pain, dyspnea, fatigue, gastrointestinal disorders, impaired cognition and mood disorders, depression, traumatic brain injuries, and sleep disorders because of the advances in genomics (Cashion, Gill, Hawes, & Henderson, 2016). The NINR has established a research agenda that focuses on improved personalized strategies to treat with precise interventions and to prevent adverse symptoms of acute and chronic illness across the continuum of care for populations in diverse settings. This is an important differentiator of the NINR strategic plan and national research agenda (Cashion & Grady, 2015; Grady, 2016).

PHARMACOGENOMICS

In addition to symptom management that occurs across many acute and chronic conditions through the continuum of care, the next largest area of all stages in the continuum of life is the area of pharmacogenomics. For example, in infancy, during attention deficit management, pain management in children and adults, clot management in cardiovascular and stroke disease, and chemotherapy, there are potentials for the patient to have genomics preventing absorption, distribution, metabolism, and elimination of drugs. The nurse can incorporate assessments and observations of adverse drug reactions resulting from pharmacogenomics in the nursing process. Variations in the human genome, specifically DNA sequence variants in enzymes, could affect a drug's ability to be used efficiently and effectively. Pharmacogenomics testing is called PGx testing, and clinical exome laboratories are cropping up across the country. Pharmacogenomics combines the science of drugs and their metabolism with genomics of enzymes that metabolize drugs to develop effective medications, safe medications, and doses tailored to the person's genetic profile. The genetic differences likely to be the most relevant in nursing assessment are those associated with genes in four broad categories: (a) genes pertinent to the drug's pharmacokinetics (PK), that is, how the person *a*bsorbs, *d*istributes, *m*etabolizes (including formation of active metabolites), and *e*xcretes a drug (ADME); (b) the pharmacodynamics (PD) of the drug, that is, how a drug affects a person; (c) genes not directly related to a drug's pharmacology that can predispose to toxicities such as immune reactions; and (d) genes that influence disease susceptibility or progression. The result is that nurses need to observe who can respond to a drug positively, who will not respond to a drug, and who will experience negative side effects called adverse drug reactions. The genomics testing in pharmacogenomics determines if it is the right drug, for the right person, at the right dose regardless of age (Collins & Varmus, 2015).

The impact of adverse drug reactions resulting from pharmacogenomics is now being studied. Adverse drug reactions cause a significant number of re-admissions to hospitals and even death. It is known that pharmacogenomics is estimated to contribute to 20% to 50% of individual drug responses in inpatients (Lea, Cheek, Brazeau, & Brazeau, 2015). The CDC estimates that more than one million emergency department visits have resulted from adverse drug reactions

(CDC, 2019). The final impact is on the cost savings of pharmacogenomics. The following are examples from a recent White Paper from Translational Software summarizing 24 studies (Relling & Evans, 2015). The cost impact of clopidogrel, an antiplatelet medication prescribed with pharmacogenomics testing, represents cost-effectiveness of $50,000 in four studies. Dramatic pharmacogenomics testing with anxiety and depression meds demonstrated an average savings of $1,800 in healthcare and $500 in medication savings per year per patient. Nine studies support the use of pharmacogenomics testing when prescribing psychiatric medications.

Further research is reported in patients over 50 and 65 years of age with polypharmacy with a potential cost savings of $1,132 to $4,400 when pharmacogenomics testing was done on these populations. Abacavir is a drug used to treat HIV/AIDS, and in some ethnic populations, a severe hypersensitivity reaction occurs and has been linked to the HLA-B*5701 allele. When pharmacogenomics testing is done to guide treatment, the cost-effectiveness per hypersensitivity reaction avoided was $26,404 per year.

The Healthcare Information and Management Systems Society (HIMSS) conducted a Precision Medicine survey in healthcare. They reported their results in 2017. The report finds that the patient's risk assessment of a patient's safety is a top issue of hospitals and vendors. Drug therapy monitoring turned out to be the second top issue of the survey (HIMSS Analytics, 2017).

Pharmacogenomics and Nursing Documentation

A preponderance of evidence for pharmacogenomics has reached sufficient evidence to incorporate into clinical practice. The NIH Pharmacogenomics Knowledge Base (PharmGKB) involves the collaboration of scientists, researchers, pharmacists, and clinicians who are collating data and disseminating information on the evidence between human genomic variation and individualized drug pharmacogenomics.

The evidence on several drug categories is published as guidelines in the Clinical Pharmacogenetics Implementation Consortium (CPIC) organization. The methods for developing these guidelines rank the level of evidence similar to clinical practice guidelines. Only those pharmacogenomics guidelines that have sufficient evidence are listed as a guideline recommended for implementation. As of December 2019, there are 150 guidelines: 47 CPIC guidelines representing the United States, 93 guidelines from the Royal Dutch Association for the Advancement of Pharmacy–Pharmacogenetics Working Group (DPWG), eight guidelines from the Canadian Pharmacogenomics Network for Drug Safety (CPNDS), and two other from professional organizations. As the consortia that recommend guidelines are continually evaluating the evidence to determine those guidelines that are sufficient, it is recommended that faculty and students visit the www.pharmgkb.org/guidelineAnnotations website regularly. There are currently 47 CPIC guidelines representing 100 drugs (PharmGKB, n.d.). Table 6.2 provides the current list of drugs and the genes regulating their metabolism. The list includes many common drugs used in clinical practice.

Table 6.2 Current List, as of December 2019, of Drugs and the Genes Regulating Their Metabolism

Drug	Gene
Abacavir	*HLA-B*
Allopurinol	*HLA-B*
Amitriptyline	*CYP2C19, CYP2D6*
Atazanavir	*UGT1A1*
Atomoxetine	*CYP2D6*
Azathioprine	*TPMT*
Capecitabine	*DPYD*
Carbamazepine	*HLA-A, HLA-B*
Citalopram	*CYP2C19*
Clomipramine	*CYP2C19, CYP2D6*
Clopidogrel	*CYP2C19*
Codeine	*CYP2D6*
Desflurane	*CACNA1S, RYR1*
Desipramine	*CYP2D6*
Doxepin	*CYP2C19, CYP2D6*
Efvirene	*CYP286*
Enflurane	*CACNA1S, RYR1*
Escitalopram	*CYP2C19*
Fluorouracil	*DPYD*
Fluvoxamine	*CYP2D6*
Halothane	*CACNA1S, RYR1*
Imipramine	*CYP2C19, CYP2D6*
Isoflurane	*CACNA1S, RYR1*
Ivacaftor	*CFTR*
Mercaptopurine	*TPMT*
Methoxyflurane	*CACNA1S, RYR1*
Nortriptyline	*CYP2D6*
Ondansetron	*CYP2D6*
Oxcarbazepine	*HLA-B*

(continued)

Table 6.2 Current List, as of December 2019, of Drugs and the Genes Regulating Their Metabolism (*continued*)

Drug	Gene
Paroxetine	*CYP2D6*
Peginterferon alfa-2a	*IFNL3*
Peginterferon alfa-2b	*IFNL3*
Phenytoin	*CYP2C9, HLA-B*
Rasburicase	*G6PD*
Ribavirin	*IFNL3*
Sertraline	*CYP2C19*
Sevoflurane	*CACNA1S, RYR1*
Simvastatin	*SLCO1B1*
Succinylcholine	*CACNA1S, RYR1*
Tacrolimus	*CYP3A5*
Tamoxifen	*CYP2D6*
Tegafur	*DPYD*
Thioguanine	*TPMT*
Trimipramine	*CYP2C19, CYP2D6*
Tropisetron	*CYP2D6*
Voriconazole	*CYP2C19*
Warfarin	*CYP2C9, CYP4F2, VKORC1*

Included in drug labeling are the variants of drugs and genetic biomarkers listed by the FDA. There are currently over 300 variants of drugs and genetic biomarkers in the queue for further international collaborative studies (FDA, 2018).

Nursing to Support Genomics With Emphasis on Symptom Management and Pharmacogenomics

There are four ways that nursing can support genomics through the nursing process. They are (a) documentation of a RAPID risk assessment; (b) family history and ethnicity; (c) medication administration and documentation; and (d) documentation evaluating medication adverse reactions (McCormick, 2017).

These were included in the July/August 2018 *Nursing Outlook* American Academy of Nursing (AAN) policy entitled "Strengthen Federal and Local Policies to Advance Precision Health Implementation and Nurses' Impact on Healthcare

Quality and Safety" (Starkweather et al., 2018). These areas can improve care quality and safety, which are also the future goals of the Quadruple Aim that leads to the improved patient experience, the enhanced clinician experience, lower costs, and better outcomes.

RAPID RISK ASSESSMENT DOCUMENTATION

Maradiegue and Edwards described the RAPID risk assessment in 2016. The **RAPID risk assessment** includes (a) assess the family history (usually recommended for at least three generations). Assess if patients or anyone in their families have had a problem metabolizing drugs. The assessment should include the information whether they were ultra-rapid metabolizers (UMs), normal or extensive metabolizers (EMs), intermediate metabolizers (IMs), or poor metabolizers (PMs), if known. (b) Identify the patient's ethnicity or ancestry, if known. (c) Establish the probability of genetic condition or predisposition to an adverse drug reaction. Consult with a geneticist, genetic counselor, or pharmacist and a physician to determine a possible adverse drug reaction or alternative drug after consulting the CPIC guideline. In the next 2 years, the number one driver of Precision Medicine in healthcare organizations is the patient risk assessment. Risk assessment is a finding in the 2017 HIMSS survey of Precision Medicine in healthcare (HIMSS Analytics, 2017).

FAMILY HISTORY IN THE NURSING ASSESSMENT DOCUMENTATION

A pedigree map or family health portrait is needed in the nursing assessment. A family health portrait should include a record of a second- and third-degree family member and his or her medical information, including age of onset of health conditions, race and ethnicity, and age and cause of death in his or her biological family. This information is becoming more readily available because, when asked, many patients have had DTC screening and ancestry tests through several online marketing tools including the cellphone. These data can identify the risks of developing common diseases and a genetic disease that runs in families. The Surgeon General of the United States Public Health Service (USPHS) recommends that during Thanksgiving dinner, each family determine the history of family illnesses to add to the family history map. A free copy of the pedigree map is available from the Health and Human Services website (https://phgkb.cdc.gov/FHH/html/index.html). Often the family learns that there are discrepancies in the results of ancestry tests, or paternity, or adoption. A conservative estimate is that in 28% to 30% of families, the man who heads the household is not the biological father (McCormick & Hoffman, 2006). When a patient shares his or her family history with nurses, often a genetics counselor, ethics counselor, or lawyers have to be brought in as consultants.

The nurse needs to record family history and ethnicity in the EHR. It has been reported in a recent study that a nursing administrator in MAGNET hospitals plays a significant role in assuring that nursing personnel have the ability to document family history and ethnicity in the EHR (Calzone, Jenkins, Culp, & Badzek, 2018).

In March 2018 at the HIMSS, two nurses from the NIH Clinical Center (CC) presented how they integrated the family history, ethnicity, and pharmacogenomics into the EHR. They are using Allscripts for their EHR with genetic testing from 2bPrecise (Wallen & Lardner, 2018). A two-pronged approach was recommended: (a) assess the limitations of the EHR for genomics and (b) evaluate the preparedness of the nurses for genomics. Their results demonstrated it was harder than they thought initially to integrate the family history into the EHR. They did succeed in implementing the family history into the EHR by stressing the importance of the role of the nurse in expanding the family history in nursing documentation to include a family history or pedigree map in the EHR. In preparing nurses for the integration into the EHR, they recommend the Method of Introducing a New Competency (MINC) implementation model. The MINC implementation model includes the following eight steps: (a) assessing nurses' genomics knowledge, (b) providing staff development, (c) providing access to assess the need to change hospital policy, (d) providing staff knowledge, (e) conducting professional development, (f) anticipating obstacles and challenges, (g) planning for integration into the EHR, and (h) educating nurses on how to use the tools (Wallen & Lardner, 2018).

ETHNICITY IN THE NURSING ASSESSMENT DOCUMENTATION

For nurses working in the United States, the population of patients in hospitals, outpatient clinics, community centers, and retail clinics can be from multiple ethnic backgrounds from around the world. The need to document ethnicity is becoming more important as we identify ethnic groups with specific diseases and deficiencies in their enzymes that metabolize drugs listed in the CPIC guidelines and are on the FDA list of biomarkers. Some specific examples will be provided in this chapter.

The average frequency of G6PD deficiency in malaria-endemic countries such as Asia and Africa is higher but varies, with a prevalence in specific population groups as high as 30% or more. For example, hemolytic anemia (AHA) and methemoglobinemia can be induced by some drugs, but especially rasburicase. It is even recommended that preemptive genotyping should be done to establish G6PD deficiency before administering rasburicase. Deficient patients are at risk of AHA, and possibly methemoglobinemia (Relling et al., 2014).

Further evidence of the need to document ethnicity is provided. It is also known that the Han Chinese, Japanese, Thai, and some Caucasians have an abnormality with the metabolism of allopurinol. The Han Chinese, Thai, Malaysians, Indians, and Japanese have enzyme deficiencies in metabolizing carbamazepine. The Han Chinese have difficulty with oxcarbazepine. The Han Chinese and Thai have metabolism issues with phenytoin. The highest risk for abacavir is in Caucasians, but risks can occur across ethnicities. The Sardinian, Japanese, Thai, and Caucasian populations have liver enzyme alleles that result in drug-induced hypersensitivity (DIHS)/drug reaction with eosinophilia system symptoms (DRESS) with a rash. The nurse can observe many of the side effects.

As previously mentioned, the patient's ethnicity is becoming more important as we examine the genetic differences in populations throughout the globe.

Table 6.3 Ethnic Variations That Nurses Should Be Aware of in Documenting Ethnicity in the Nursing Assessment

Site	Conditions/Disease
Luxembourg (Centre for Systems Biomedicine)	Parkinson's disease
Singapore (POLARIS)	Pilot *TGFBI* testing for disease diagnosis and family risk assessment in stromal corneal dystrophies and gastrointestinal cancers
Sri Lanka	Thalassemia carriers and genetic modifiers to convert thalassemia to manageable, chronic illness
Thailand (Pharmacogenomics and Personalized Medicine)	The risk for drugs with risk for Stevens–Johnson syndrome/toxic epidermal necrolysis

Source: Manolio, T. A., Abramawiz, M., Al-Mulla, F., Anderson, W., Balling, R., Berger, A. C., … Leego, E. (2015). Global implementation of genomic medicine: We are not alone. *Science Translational Medicine, 7*(290), 290–303. doi:10.1126/scitranslmed.aab0194

Table 6.3 identifies some of those ethnic variations that the genomic studies internationally are disclosing (Manolio et al., 2015).

Nursing's Role in Medication Administration and Documentation

Nursing has a professional standard and licensure requirements to document medication administration. Previously, the standards charged nurses with five rights: the right patient, right dose, right drug, right route, and the right time. Today, with the CPIC guideline implementation and the foundation of pharmacogenomics in Precision Health in diverse ethnic populations, it is the *right drug, for the right person, at the right dose regardless of age* (Collins & Varmus, 2015). The number two driver of change required in the future for hospitals and vendors is drug therapy monitoring according to the 2017 HIMSS survey of Precision Medicine in healthcare organizations (HIMSS Analytics, 2017).

Evaluation of Medication Adverse Reactions

Box 6.2 lists the most frequent adverse toxic events to drugs. The list of adverse reactions is an expanded list of adverse medication reactions from the previous publication in 2017 (McCormick, 2017).

Box 6.2 Listing of Frequent Adverse Toxic Events to Drugs

Anemia
Bone marrow hypocellular
Disseminated intravascular coagulation
Febrile neutropenia
Hemolysis
Hemolytic uremic syndrome
Leukocytosis
Lymph node pain
Spleen disorder
Thrombocytopenic thrombotic purpura
Skin irritations such as exanthema, urticaria, and angioedema
Severe cutaneous adverse reactions
Stevens–Johnson syndrome
Toxic epidermal necrosis
Drug-induced hypersensitivity
Drug reaction with eosinophilia system symptoms
Nausea, vomiting, diarrhea, and stomach pain
Myopathy
Cough, shortness of breath, and sore throat
Thrombus/clots
Nose bleeds
Hematuria

In the current environment, nurses require access to additional information and expertise in evaluating the impact of adverse medication reactions. The three examples of drugs on the CPIC guideline list and the drug reactions are as follows: (a) Drug hypersensitivity remains an important clinical issue in evaluating syndromes such as abacavir hypersensitivity reaction, allopurinol DRESS/DIHS and Stevens–Johnson syndrome/toxic epidermal necrolysis (SJS/TEN), and SJS/TEN associated with aromatic amine anticonvulsants. (b) Clopidogrel is a platelet adenosine diphosphate (ADP)–receptor antagonist that is indicated for the reduction of atherothrombotic events in patients with recent myocardial infarction, recent stroke, peripheral artery disease, and acute coronary syndrome. Case Study 6.1 discusses the nurse's role in monitoring clopidogrel. (c) Warfarin is a Coumadin-based anticoagulant that is widely used for the short- and long-term management of thromboembolic disorders, such as deep-vein thrombosis, and is used to prevent stroke and systemic embolic events in patients with atrial fibrillation and those undergoing orthopedic surgeries. A relatively large number of patients experience life-threatening bleeding complications from warfarin. It has been consistently a top 10-ranked cause of drug-induced serious adverse reactions. Nose bleeds and blood in the urine are reported relatively frequently. Underlying genetic factors have been shown to account for approximately 35% to 40% of the variation in the maintenance dose.

CASE STUDY 6.1

THE STORY OF VICTORIA: PHARMACOGENOMICS—CLOPIDOGREL AND PRASUGREL

Victoria is a 68-year-old woman with hypertension, hyperlipidemia, and severe peripheral artery disease (PAD) of both legs who lives with minimal assistance in an older adult residence. She was admitted to the emergency department (ED) with shortness of breath and profound weakness. Diagnostic studies confirmed a myocardial infarction (MI). Upon cardiac catheterization, a 95% left anterior descending coronary artery occlusion was managed with a single intracoronary artery stent. After several days, she was discharged with most of her prehospital medications; however, clopidogrel (Plavix), her previously prescribed antiplatelet drug, was stopped, and a new agent, prasugrel (Effient), was prescribed.

When Victoria filled the new drug at her community retail clinic and pharmacy, she learned the new drug was $81 for a month, compared to $10 per month for clopidogrel. She asked the nurse practitioner to continue her clopidogrel prescription. Victoria has a 1-week supply left and will take it. Jean, the nurse practitioner, called the cardiologist who said that Victoria developed an intracoronary artery thrombosis on clopidogrel. The cardiologist further stated that as many as 20% of patients do not receive benefit from clopidogrel. Jean scheduled a pharmacogenomics test to determine Victoria's profile and address concerns about the selection of an effective drug. The pharmacogenomics test was paid for by Medicare (http://cms.hhs.gov) since it included an analysis of *nine* common cytochrome P450 (CYP) enzymes involved in drug metabolism. The pharmacogenomics test revealed Victoria was a slow CYP2C19 metabolizer. The result confirmed clopidogrel was unlikely to be effective in a reduced antiplatelet response and ineffective in the prevention of further thrombosis after stent procedures. A prodrug is a medication that needs to be converted to an active form. Metabolism of drugs occurs through metabolism in the liver. Typically, slow metabolizers do not convert sufficient quantities of clopidogrel to an active antiplatelet agent; slow metabolizers of clopidogrel are at an increased risk of cardiovascular events after stent placement (Price, 2012). The FDA estimates that 2% to 14% of patients are poor metabolizers of clopidogrel. Prasugrel is an active drug that is deactivated by CYP3A4 and 2B6 enzymes, with minor involvement of the 2C19 enzymes (FDA, 2016). Because Victoria's pharmacogenomics tests revealed no concerns about 2B6, Jean noted that prasugrel (Effient) is likely to be more effective.

This change and issue with metabolism were not explained to Victoria in the hospital, including why she was changed to a new drug. The hospital did not do the pharmacogenomics test for her enzyme. An interoperable EHR or personal health record (PHR) would have communicated across settings why the cardiologist prescribed prasugrel in the hospital upon discharge and would have added to the cardiologist's knowledge of other patients that may have the inability to metabolize clopidogrel in the liver.

Because she was concerned about the costs, Jean contacted the manufacturer of the drug and they successfully enrolled Victoria in a program to decrease her out-of-pocket expenses. Victoria registered for cardiac rehabilitation, recovered uneventfully, and experienced no complications from severe PAD on her new antiplatelet regime. As her retail clinic primary care nurse, Jean's knowledge of pharmacology and pharmacogenomics ensured Victoria's care was personalized (precise), and outcomes were met to reflect quality patient care.

LINKING GENOMICS AND BIOINFORMATICS

Figure 6.1 is the modern-day graphical representation of the knowledge and skills required to integrate the science of genomics with the computational skills (Bioinformatics) needed to analyze these data. This figure has been adapted from a publication by Regan et al. (2018) in the *Journal of Nursing Scholarship* that focused on the OMICS (genomics, proteomics, transcriptomics, and metabolomics). The original figure in this chapter integrates the elements of genomics with the bioinformatics needs from populations to Precision Health and individual or personal health.

Unique Needs for Security

As the personal information of the individual includes his or her genomics linked to his or her phenotype (how a person's genes, biology, and environment come together to make up a person), the security of these data become a pinnacle test of a person's willingness to participate in the Precision Health that can benefit his or her diagnosis and treatment. The issues regarding the security surrounding this occur within entire sections of books, and this author recommends the section by Dr. Dixie Baker in *Healthcare Information Technology* (Baker, 2018).

Implementation Using Digital Tools and Promoting Integration of Genomics and Pharmacogenomics Guidelines Into the EHR

Previous papers have described various efforts in the United States to develop road maps toward the integration of genomics and pharmacogenomics guidelines into the EHR. Recent advances include St. Jude's Hospital, whose staff developed a model workflow and computer decision support (CDS) for incorporating genomics and pharmacogenomics tests into the EHR (Hoffman et al., 2014).

Several NIH-supported initiatives have translational research efforts to Implement Genomics in Practice (a project called IGNITE). There are six participating research sites in this program—the University of Florida, Duke University (which also serves as the coordinating center), Icahn School of Medicine at Mount Sinai, Vanderbilt University, University of Maryland, and Indiana University coordinated by the NHGRI (NHGRI, 2019c). This consortium of universities has produced customized implementation tools (SPARK toolbox) for some of the CPIC guidelines. The information is helpful for developers and clinicians implementing the CPIC guidelines.

Another translational research effort is called the Electronic Medical Records and Genomics (eMERGE) Network. The eMERGE Network is organized and funded by the NIH. The research centers combine DNA biorepositories with electronic medical record (EMR) systems for large-scale, high-throughput genetic research in support of implementing genomics. The eMERGE Network members (as of November 2019) are Brigham and Women's Hospital with Massachusetts General Hospital, Cincinnati Children's Hospital Medical Center and Boston Children's Hospital, Children's Hospital of Philadelphia, Columbia University, Geisinger, Kaiser Permanente Washington, Marshfield Clinic, Mayo Clinic, Meharry Medical College, Mount Sinai School of Medicine, Northwestern

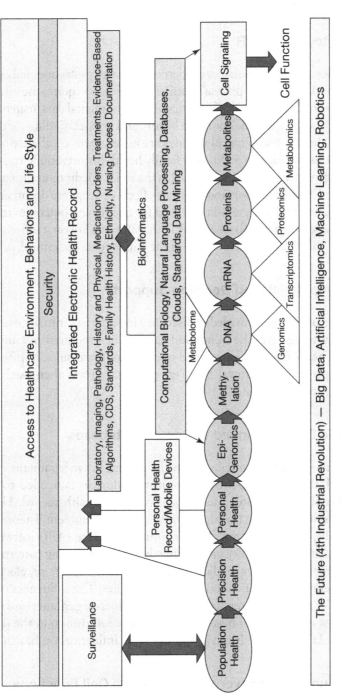

Figure 6.1 Relationship between OMICS science and informatics.

CDS, computer decision support.

Source: Manolio, T. A., Abramowiz, M., Al-Mulla, F., Anderson, W., Balling, R., Berger, A. C., ... Leego, E. (2015). Global implementation of genomic medicine: We are not alone. *Science Translational Medicine, 7*(290), 290–303. doi:10.1126/scitranslmed.aab0194

University, and Vanderbilt University. The coordinating center is at Vanderbilt University, and the Brigham and Women's Hospital with the Broad Institute and Baylor College of Medicine serve as the sequencing and genotyping facilities (NHGRI, 2019a).

The Need for the Integrated EHR

The combination of the gene sequencing process through proteomics and cell function leading to the diagnosis and precise treatment of diseases requires the integration of large volumes of data from bioinformatics, to environmental data, matched to large population databases, and the complete history and physical findings of the patient. The person's history and physical findings are necessary to combine with imaging data and laboratory data. In addition, a family health history, ethnicity, and risk assessment of genomic potential are needed in the EHR. Medication administration is posted in the EHR, and observations of side effects of drugs are documented in the EHR. Evaluation and analyses of these data for quality and outcomes require new tools with these integrated databases. Whether the data are on stand-alone servers or in clouds, the security and integrity of the patient data are critical.

Algorithms and Computer-Based Decision Support

Data mining and simple knowledge discovery in databases initially used a variety of algorithms to discover the trends and patterns in structured and unstructured databases. Then tools were developed to compare the results in different databases. Text processing (natural language processing) was then used to extract data from unstructured data.

The Need for Mobile Devices Linked to Secure Databases

Because so much data are attributed to the patient in environments other than the hospital, the use of electronic monitoring devices is needed to integrate with the hospital, ambulatory EHR, and personal health record. Homes will be connected in the future through cameras, sensors, ambient listening devices, Internet hubs, and Application Programming Interface (API) software. Some other devices include mobility monitoring, heart rate, smoking patterns, alcohol, drug use, over-the-counter medications, level of stress, exercise, electrocardiogram, temperature, weight, blood pressure, and diet. The influences of these on metabolomics and environmental factors can influence genomes and the effects of treatments on diseases. These were previously referred to in the description of Precision Health as the lifestyle and behavior influences on health.

Bioinformatics to Support Discovery of Genetics to Cell Functions

To discover genes, their function, and variation, bioinformatics tools are needed. Bioinformatics is the branch of biology that is concerned with the acquisition, storage, and display and analysis of the information found in nucleic acid and protein sequence data (NHGRI, n.d.-a).

Chip-based science, microarray technology and analytics, and next-generation sequencing have led the field of the discovery of genes. Genome sequencing uncovers the specific order of the DNA building blocks (ATCG). High throughput has allowed the sequencing of DNA to occur in a single day—a process that took a decade 25 years ago. Techniques in molecular genetics, combined with robust statistical and epidemiology approaches, have produced gene–environment interactions. Correlating the molecular response with the environment allows us to recognize persons who have a susceptibility to a genetic alteration who may not lead to disease because of environmental factors. Expansion of information at the molecular level has led to large databases kept by the NIH to detect variations in a gene's sequence for multiple diseases. The volume of discoveries from gene sequencing and proteomics is necessitating AI.

Database support: The large volumes of data produced from the gene require databases capable of supporting the data. Comparative and population data add to the enormous database support needed to determine variations by communities, environmental differences, clinical trial responses, and surveillance data. Initially, the databases that were built used advanced data mining analytics. Today, the data have to be put into clouds to support the enormous volume of data. Through the security of clouds, the data can be accessible with new standards sharing APIs and Fast Healthcare Interoperability Resources (FHIR).

Moving to AI, ML, Big Data Clouds, and Robotics

The volume of data represented in Case Study 6.1 and Figure 6.1 is Big Data. Genomics for one individual results in about 1 TB of data (McCormick & Calzone, 2016). When sequencing is performed on one individual, the exome analysis alone results in 6 to 8 GB of data. Whole-genome sequencing generates between 100 and 200 GB of data. That number does not include the volume of data resulting from history and physical, imaging data, laboratory data, clinical observations, tissue biopsy results, morphology, or the multiple times that data genomics tests and imaging data have to be redone during radiation and/or drug treatment.

Algorithms developed by humans and learned by computers are the basic foundation for ML. Thanks to the integration of data through clouds and the Internet, the volume of data now requires new technologies to read, analyze, and process it, as well as recommend linkages in information, thus converting it to knowledge. It is through these steps that the machine can learn. This new knowledge can be the basis for new decisions to support diagnosis, treatment, imaging, and other tests for AI and ML. The volume of data has exceeded the abilities of the entire clinical team (nurses, doctors, pharmacists, geneticists) to process the digital information for a single patient, let alone large groups of patients, extrapolated to the population.

In the past, groups of patients were looked at through statistical methods, sampling, and linear regression to predict outcomes of care. The science has evolved to enabling artificial neural networks. Computer models are possible and artificial neural networks are capable of carrying out data task identification to match information and describe the relationship between them.

Because these networks can be stored, the network is capable of changing and adapting to the analyses of data passing through it. Through this process, it can "learn," based upon data alone, and devoid of interpretations and judgments. These networks can be passed through concurrent pathways of complex algorithms to enable analyses of complete pathways and the results provided to the clinical team. That is where the clinician is provided the information for clinical decision-making.

Already under development are new platforms to integrate and analyze the data from all of these elements to make a decision on the cell. One project called the Baseline from Verily is a longitudinal study being conducted at Duke University and Stanford. This project collects data across clinical, molecular, imaging, sensor, self-reported, behavioral, psychological, environmental, and other health-related measurements from onsite visits, continuous data collection through sensor technology, and regular engagement via an online portal and mobile applications. With integrated data, it is expected that scientists will be able to analyze the data to provide a range of expected values among a diverse population and provide biomarkers of cardiovascular and cancer disease-related transitions.

AI AND ROBOTICS IN GENOMICS

The promise of imaging and sensory technology AI and ML are being applied to genomic data to help understand and predict the diagnosis and treatment of cancer, how cancer spreads, and the importance of the integration of genomics with transcriptomics, proteomics, and metabolomics. The underlying function of cells in the membrane of cancer tumors offers new promise for applications in AI and ML. The ultimate goals of AI and ML are to describe the genome of a single person, to determine the best drug therapies, based on the DNA of the person's healthy cells and tumors. Embedded in this analysis is the number of mutations that the person has that require analysis of the impact of the mutation and the pathway that the abnormal cells will metastasize (spread). Also, sequencing of genes has evolved from cumbersome and time-consuming technology to rapid next-generation sequencing and the use of robots to process genetic sequences. There are many more applications of robotics in healthcare, but they are beyond the scope of this chapter.

CHALLENGES

Reimbursement to Assure Access to Personalized Health and Clinical Implementation

The first FDA-approved diagnostic testing with Medicare coverage included all solid tumors, including NSCLC, colorectal, breast, ovarian, and melanoma.

By 2018, the Centers for Medicare & Medicaid Services (CMS) reimbursed 324 genes and two genomic signatures in any solid tumor so that therapies could be targeted. CMS took action to advance innovative personalized medicine for Medicare patients with cancer (FDA, 2017b). These websites need to be monitored routinely because CMS National Coverage Determinations have recently been subject to change. Without CMS coverage, the patient and research costs will have to pay for genomic tests.

At this time, all the regions covered by CMS Medicare Administrative Contractors (MACs) are currently reimbursing for the following: CYP2C19 for patients undergoing PCI or clopidogrel therapy, CYP2D6 for therapy with amitriptyline/nortriptyline (for depression) or tetrabenazine, CYP2C for warfarin treatment in anticoagulation, and VKORC1 for anticoagulation therapy (https://www.cms.gov/Regulations-and-Guidance/Guidance/Transmittals/2018Downloads/R3999CP.pdf).

Educating Nurses With Enough Clinical Knowledge and Expertise in the Era of Precision Health

Initial training focused on computer-aided instruction to train those not highly trained in bioinformatics. The needs became magnified when the translation of genetic and genomic discoveries was being applied in clinical practice. Leaders in the field of training and the development of competencies were the NHGRI, the NLM, the National Cancer Institute (NCI), the FDA, the Department of Energy (DOE), and the National Institute of Standards and Technology (NIST). These remain legitimate training areas for the fields of bioinformatics and genomics.

The rapidity of discoveries and uptake of genetics into society drive the need for more competent educated nurses in academia, practice, research, and education. The AAN policy entitled "Strengthen Federal and Local Policies to Advance Precision Health Implements and Nurses' Impact on Healthcare Quality and Safety" (Starkweather et al., 2018) recommends sufficient education and continuing education on implementing Precision Health, and the integration of data sources into the information technology infrastructure to provide clinical support for healthcare providers to document a RAPID risk assessment, ethnicity, and family history; to include CPIC guidelines for clinicians; computerized decision supports; and the ability to document adverse drug reactions. Clinicians will have to be educated about how to deliver genomic information to nurses, doctors, geneticists, genetic counselors, pharmacists, and patients. New tools are being developed and tested in several academic centers throughout the country. Some of the tools to follow are SimulConsult funded by the NIH, decision support from the eMERGE Network, InfoButtons, Compass Gene Report, CLEAR and CASCADE Chatbots, and Monitored Frequently Asked Question Sites on mobile applications.

Ethical and Legal Challenges

There are four challenges to moving forward with nursing and genomics. The first is privacy and the attempts to balance consulting research and protecting genetic information. The second is regulations that protect patients and data, and the balance with innovation.

The third is assuring against discrimination, which has been addressed by the Genetic Information Nondiscrimination Act of 2008 (referred to as GINA). The final is fraud and abuse with free or reduced-cost testing allowances. The challenges in ethics and laws are resulting from the advances in genetic testing and technological advances such as gene editing.

Privacy is important because your genome is more personal than your fingerprint. It says what your health status is and risk for diseases. Where the data are stored and how secure the sequence banks are creates another area of privacy. Using the data for law enforcement has become a large media-covered use of genomics.

Using sequencing data for research by other researchers is another privacy issue because the person consenting may not have consented for additional researchers to use the data.

The current legal framework for protecting the privacy of genomic data is the Health Insurance Portability and Accountability Act (HIPAA), which currently allows the use of data for research and allows sharing de-identified data. The interpretation of HIPAA and the definition of research may vary by states. The Office of Human Research Protections (OHRP) at HHS protects human subjects.

Even though we have the GINA of 2008 as a federal law that was enacted to prevent discrimination in health insurers and employers based on genetic and genomic information, consumers remain fearful of genetic discrimination. Ten years after GINA was passed, it is recognized that the current law does not include military personnel, nor does it cover persons acquiring life insurance, disability insurance, and long-term care insurance. The AAN policy on strengthening federal and local policies to advance Precision Health implementation recommends enhancements to the HIPAA and GINA that are appropriate to Precision Health implementation (Starkweather et al., 2018). Generally, any genetic treatments or technologies that enhance the human are considered unethical.

New cases of genetic malpractice are coming into existence, and the majority could have been avoided if genetic testing had been performed. Few cases exist where genetic testing led to the wrong diagnosis and resulted in the mismanagement of the patient's diagnosis or treatment. The nursing professionals representing policy committees and advocacy groups of professional organizations need to remain vigilant monitoring the policies and laws governing genetics and genomic data that protect the healthcare consumers. They need to respond to draft documents on ethical challenges in genetics and genomics.

The Challenge of Nursing Culture

According to Francis Collins and his AI Working Group, we are entering into a fourth Industrial Revolution (Glazer & Tabak, 2018). Genetics and genomics discoveries and the volume of data produced by them are driving the needs for Big Data, robotics, clouds, AI, and ML. The integration of genetic and genomic data into EHRs and the integration of the genomics with measurements of lifestyle and behaviors, the environment, and access to care are creating needs for innovative information technology solutions. These are the forces described in Table 6.1 that separate Precision Medicine from Precision Health. These forces are compelling a cultural shift in the way we integrate data from many sources to look at the patient as an n-of-1, in addition to looking at health from a population perspective of groups of patients. These forces are expanding our thinking beyond diagnosis and treatment to include prevention and symptom management. New nursing observations in patient care need to include the RAPID risk assessment, family history, ethnicity, medication administration, and documentation. Evaluation of medication adverse reactions becomes a part of the new culture of Precision Health. The cultural advances require the nursing profession to change our DNA to include genomics in our care to patients. By changing nursing's DNA to a culture of care using genomics, the nursing profession will provide enormous opportunities for nurses to improve the quality and outcomes of care and improve patient safety. Nurses have always been early adopters of new technology and changes in healthcare. The patient is moving quickly into accepting genetics and genomics as evidenced by the number of DTC tests being performed. To remain in the most trusted profession, nurses need to embrace the culture changes in Precision Health.

Currently, the entire genome is too large to store in an EHR, so external databases in clouds linked to the EHR are alternatives being explored. An EHR system vendor, Epic, has implemented "Genomic Indicators" in their clinical record system and allows CDS around genomic variants. The new HL7 FHIR is also working as a member of a consortium (agile genomics) to get data into the EHR. There are also not enough clinicians in medicine, nursing, genetic counseling, or genetics, or pharmacists, to handle large-scale sequencing. Another barrier to utilizing genomics in healthcare is the already complex clinical workflow and regulatory demands. New genomic practice guidelines, in addition to the CPIC guidelines, are needed to inform nurses what genetic results are ready for implementation into practice and how to manage all the patient's genetic test results.

Nursing to Support Genomics in the Future

The key technology to going forward toward Precision Health will be a challenge to integrate the necessary information for nursing assessment, documentation, and assessment of outcomes into the EHR. Integration of genomic data into the EHR for patient management and decision support is critical to enable nurses to practice Precision Health. Bridging the daily living of patients with their outpatient visits and hospitalizations will remain a priority. Even patient visits to retail clinics will have to be integrated into patient record systems. Networks of health information include enormous amounts of data that require additional security, unique patient identifiers, and CDS tools. AI and analytics will be needed to evaluate the quality and outcomes of these Big Data.

Of all the advantages of Precision Health to nursing, hypothetically the most valuable will be in prevention, risk assessment, symptom management, and pharmacogenomics. Prevention, risk assessment, symptom management, and pharmacogenomics will require closer collaboration with genetic nurse counselors and pharmacists, in addition to medical colleagues and geneticists. The genetic nurse counselors and pharmacists, in addition to medical colleagues and geneticists, are the new team in the tumor boards, because of the molecular nature of the diseases. Genomics is quickly becoming an integral part of healthcare practice.

In the future, nurses will individually be able to identify genes that inform patients what diseases they are likely to have as they get older. The genes will be able to inform nurses how patients will react to medications; how they will respond to infectious diseases; how wounds will heal; how they tolerate pain, sleep, and what to eat; and how to exercise.

In the HIMSS Analytics (2017) survey of Precision Medicine in healthcare (previously mentioned), providers identified their top three challenges to implementing Precision Medicine initiatives. Those challenges, in order of significance, were identified as (a) budget and financial reasons, (b) issues integrating clinical and genomic data into current systems, and (c) lack of clinical knowledge or expertise.

CONCLUSION

By the time this chapter goes to print and the reader digests where we have been and where we have the potential to go with technologies, the giants in technology (Google, Amazon, Apple, and Facebook) will be translating all of the integrating healthcare information and advanced communication strategies to our smartphones. IBM will continue to develop the necessary components of engineering, models, and tools for enhancing the capabilities of natural language processing, voice (speech) and image recognition, and reasoning. They are seeking to create smarter, more useful technology to incentivize personal medicine.

Also, by the time this chapter goes to print, a new book titled *Deep Medicine: How Artificial Intelligence Can Make Healthcare Human Again*, by Dr. Eric Topol (2019), will also be out. In the book, Eric Topol suggests that advances in AI will improve the accuracy of diagnosis and treatment in disease.

GLOSSARY

Genetics: The study of individual genes and their impact on relatively rare single-gene disorders.

Genomics: The study of all the genes in the human genome together, including their interactions with each other, their environment, and other psychosocial and cultural factors.

OMICS: The study of genomics, proteomics, transcriptomics, and metabolomics.

Pharmacogenomics: A branch of pharmacology concerned with using DNA and amino acid sequence data to inform drug development and testing. An important application of pharmacogenomics is correlating individual genetic variation with drug responses.

Precision Health: An emerging approach for disease treatment and prevention that takes into account individual variability in genes, environment, and lifestyle for each person.

RAPID Risk Assessment: Includes (a) assess the family history (usually recommended for at least three generations), (b) identify the patient's ethnicity or ancestry, if known, and (c) establish the probability of genetic condition or predisposition to an adverse drug reaction.

THOUGHT-PROVOKING QUESTIONS

1. Should nurses research the adverse reactions to all drugs in the CPIC guidelines?

2. What is the next generation of nursing policies that should be developed to support genomics?

3. If nursing manages the lifestyle and behaviors, symptom management, and genomics, is the profession engaged in the significant components of health in the population?

4. Should the quality impact of adverse reactions and rehospitalizations be evaluated in hospitals for quality assurance by external auditors?

5. Should the economic impact of adverse reactions and not matching the genomics of diagnosis and prognosis with treatment be evaluated by nurse managers and hospital administrators?

REFERENCES

American Nurses Association. (2010). *ANA's principles for nursing documentation: Guidance for registered nurses*. Silver Spring, MD: Author.

American Nurses Association. (2015). *Nursing informatics: Scope and standards of practice* (2nd ed.). Silver Spring, MD: Author.

Baker, D. B. (2018). Framework for privacy, security, and confidentiality. In K. A. McCormick, B. Gugerty, & J. E. Mattison (Eds.), *Healthcare information technology exam, guide for CHTS and caHIMSS* (pp. 639–669). New York, NY: McGraw-Hill Education.

Calzone, K. A., Jenkins, J., Culp, S., & Badzek, L. (2018). Hospital nursing leadership-led interventions increased genomic awareness and educational intent in Magnet settings. *Nursing Outlook, 66*, 244–253. doi:10.1016/j.outlook.2017.10.010

Cashion, A. K., & Grady, P. A. (2015). The National Institutes of Health/National Institute of Nursing Research Intramural Research Program and the development of the National Institutes of Health Symptom Science Model. *Nursing Outlook, 63*(4), 484–487.

Cashion, A. K., Gill, J., Hawes, R., & Henderson, W. A. (2016). The National Institutes of Health Symptom Science Model sheds light on patient symptoms. *Nursing Outlook, 64*(5), 499–506.

Centers for Disease Control and Prevention. (2018, February). *World birth defects day*. Retrieved from https://www.cdc.gov/features/birth-defects-day/index.html

Centers for Disease Control and Prevention. (2019). *Medication safety program: Program focus*. Retrieved from https://www.cdc.gov/medicationsafety/program_focus_activities.html

Collins, F. S., & Varmus, H. (2015). Perspective: New initiative on Precision Medicine. *New England Journal of Medicine, 372*, 793–795. doi:10.1056/NEJMp1500523

Genetic and Rare Diseases Information Center. (2018). *NLM rare diseases 2000 and 2,938 articles effectiveness disease and drug studies*. Retrieved from https://rarediseases.info.nih.gov

Glazer, D., & Tabak, L. A. (2018, December 14). *Artificial Intelligence Working Group update*. 117th Meeting of the Advisory Committee to the Director (ACD). Retrieved from https://acd.od.nih.gov/documents/presentations/12142018AI.pdf

Grady, P. A. (2016). *NINR strategic plan*. Retrieved from https://www.ninr.nih.gov/sites/files/docs/NINR_StratPlan2016_reduced.pdf

Guttmacher, A. E., Collins, F. S., & Drazen, J. M. (2004). *Genomic medicine—Articles from the New England Journal of Medicine*. Baltimore, MD: The Johns Hopkins University Press.

Health Resources and Services Administration. (2019). *Recommended uniform screening panel: Core conditions*. Retrieved from https://www.hrsa.gov/sites/default/files/hrsa/advisory-committees/heritable-disorders/rusp/rusp-uniform-screening-panel.pdf

HIMSS Analytics. (2017). *2017 precision medicine study*. Retrieved from https://www.definitivehc.com/resources/essential-brief/2017-precision-medicine-study

Hoffman, J. M., Haidar, C. E., Wilkinson, M. R., Crews, K. R., Baker, D. K., Kornegay, N. M., ... Relling, M. V. (2014). PG4KDS: A model for the clinical implementation of pre-emptive pharmacogenetics. *American Journal of Medical Genetics C: Seminars in Medical Genetics*, *166C*(1), 45–55. doi:10.1002/ajmg.c.31391

Kaplan, M., & Hammerman, C. (2008, July). Neonatal hyperbilirubinemia: Don't let glucose-6-phosphate dehydrogenase deficiency off the hook. *Pediatrics*, *122*(1), 217–218. doi:10.1542/peds.2008-0834

Lea, D. H., Cheek, D., Brazeau, D., & Brazeau, G. (2015). *Mastering pharmacogenomics: A nurse's handbook for success*. Indianapolis, IN: Sigma Theta Tau.

Manolio, T. A., Abramawiz, M., Al-Mulla, F., Anderson, W., Balling, R., Berger, A. C., ... Leego, E. (2015). Global implementation of genomic medicine: We are not alone. *Science Translational Medicine*, *7*(290), 290–303. doi:10.1126/scitranslmed.aab0194

Maradiegue, A. H., & Edwards, Q. T. (2016). A primer: Risk assessment, data collection, and interpretation for genomic clinical assessment. In D. C. Siebert, Q. T. Edwards, A. H. Maradiegue, & S. T. Tinley (Eds.), *Genomic essentials for graduate level nurses* (pp. 31–66). Lancaster, PA: DEStech Publications.

McCormick, K. A. (2017). Together into the future ... Pharmacogenomics and documentation. *Nursing Management*, *48*, 32–40. doi:10.1097/01.NUMA.0000515793.26355.7f

McCormick, K. A., & Calzone, K. A. (2016). The impact of genomics on health outcomes, quality and safety. *Nursing Management*, *47*(4), 23–26. doi:10.1097/01.NUMA.0000481844.50047.ee

McCormick, K. A., & Hoffman, M. (2006). Influence of biomedical informatics on clinical information systems. In C. Weaver, C. Delaney, P. Weber, & R. Carr (Eds.), *Nursing and informatics for the 21st century: Cases, practice, and the future* (pp. 473–482). Chicago, IL: HIMSS Press.

MD Anderson Cancer Center. (2018). *Long-term IMPACT data find improved survival when targeted therapies matched to tumor-specific gene mutations.* Retrieved from https://www.mdanderson.org/newsroom/2018/05/long-term-impact-data-find-improved-survival-when-targeted-therapies-matched-to-tumor-specific-gene-mutations.html

National Center for Biotechnology Information, U.S. National Library of Medicine. (n.d.-a). *ClinVar*. Retrieved from https://www.ncbi.nlm.nih.gov/clinvar

National Center for Biotechnology Information, U.S. National Library of Medicine. (n.d.-b). *dbGaP*. Retrieved from https://www.ncbi.nlm.nih.gov/gap

National Human Genome Research Institute. (n.d.-a). Talking glossary of genetic terms: Bioinformatics. Retrieved from https://www.genome.gov/genetics-glossary/Bioinformatics

National Human Genome Research Institute. (n.d.-b). Talking glossary of genetic terms: Genomics. Retrieved from https://www.genome.gov/genetics-glossary/genomics

National Human Genome Research Institute. (n.d.-c). Talking glossary of genetic terms: Pharmacogenomics. Retrieved from https://www.genome.gov/genetics-glossary/Pharmacogenomics

National Human Genome Research Institute. (2019a). *Electronic Medical Records and Genomics (eMERGE) Network*. Retrieved from https://www.genome.gov/Funded-Programs-Projects/Electronic-Medical-Records-and-Genomics-Network-eMERGE

National Human Genome Research Institute. (2019b). *The cost of sequencing a human genome*. Retrieved from https://www.genome.gov/27565109/the-cost-of-sequencing-a-human-genome

National Human Genome Research Institute. (2019c). *Implementing Genomics in Practice (IGNITE)*. Retrieved from https://www.genome.gov/Funded-Programs-Projects/Implementing-Genomics-in-Practice-IGNITE

National Institutes of Health. (2018). *TAILORx trial finds most women with early breast cancer do not benefit from chemotherapy*. Retrieved from https://www.nih.gov/news-events/news-releases/tailorx-trial-finds-most-women-early-breast-cancer-do-not-benefit-chemotherapy

National Institutes of Health All of Us Research Program. (2017). *The future of health begins with you*. Retrieved from https://allofus.nih.gov

PharmGKB. (n.d.). *Clinical guideline annotations—CPIC*. Retrieved from https://www.pharmgkb.org/guidelineAnnotations

Phillips, K. A., Deverka, P. A., & Hooker, G. W. (2018). Genetic test availability and spending: Where are we now? Where are we going? *Health Affairs, 27*(4), 710–716. doi:10.1377/hlthaff.2017.1427

Price, M. J. (2012). Genetic considerations. *Advances in Cardiology, 47*, 100–113. doi:10.1159/000338043

Regan, M., Engler, M. B., Coleman, B., Daack-Hirsch, S., & Calzone, K. A. (2018). Establishing the genomic knowledge matrix for nursing science. *Journal of Nursing Scholarship, 51*, 50–57. doi:10.1111/jnu,12427

Relling, M. V., & Evans, W. E. (2015). Pharmacogenomics in the clinic. *Nature, 526*(7573), 343–350. doi:10.1038/nature15817

Relling, M. V., McDonagh, E. M., Chang, R., Caudle, K. E., McLeod, H. L., Haidar, C. E., ... Luzzatto, L. (2014). Clinical Pharmacogenetics Implementation Consortium (CPIC) guidelines for rasburicase therapy in the context of G6PD deficiency genotype. *Clinical Pharmacology and Therapeutics, 96*(2), 169–174. doi:10.1038/clpt.2014.97

Ridley, M. (1999). *Genome: The autobiography of species in 23 chapters*. New York, NY: HarperCollins Publishers.

Schroeder, S. A. (2007). We can do better—Improving the health of the American people. *New England Journal of Medicine, 357*, 1221–1228. doi:10.1056/NEJMsa073350

Shrestha, R. (2018). The rise in genomics in healthcare. *Healthcare Leadership Blog*. Retrieved from https://hcldr.wordpress.com/2018/04/11/the-rise-of-genomics-in-health-care

Starkweather, A. R., Coleman, B., Barcelona de Mendoza, V., Hickey, K., Menzies, V., Fu, M., ... Harper, E. (2018). Strengthen federal and local policies to advance precision health implementation and nurses' impact on healthcare quality and safety. *Nursing Outlook, 66*, 401–406. doi:10.1016/j.outlook.2018.06.001

Topol, E. (2019, March 12). *Deep medicine: How artificial intelligence can make healthcare human again*. New York, NY: Basic Books.

21st Century Cures Act. (2016). *Public law 114–255: 114th Congress*. Retrieved from https://www.congress.gov/114/plaws/publ255/PLAW-114publ255.pdf

U.S. Food and Drug Administration. (2016, September). *FDA drug safety communication: Reduced effectiveness of Plavix (clopidogrel) in patients who are poor metabolizers*. Retrieved from https://www.fda.gov/drugs/postmarket-drug-safety-information-patients-and-providers/fda-drug-safety-communication-reduced-effectiveness-plavix-clopidogrel-patients-who-are-poor

U.S. Food and Drug Administration. (2017a). *FDA allows marketing of first direct-to-consumer tests that provide genetic risk information for certain conditions*. Retrieved from https://www.fda.gov/newsevents/newsroom/pressannouncements/ucm551185.htm

U.S. Food and Drug Administration. (2017b, November 30). *FDA announces approval, CMS proposes coverage of first breakthrough-designated test to detect an extensive number of cancer biomarkers*. Retrieved from https://www.fda.gov/newsevents/newsroom/pressannouncements/ucm587273.htm

U.S. Food and Drug Administration. (2018). *Table of pharmacogenomic biomarkers in drug labeling*. Retrieved from https://www.fda.gov/downloads/Drugs/ScienceResearch/UCM578588.pdf

Wallen, G., & Lardner, M. (2018, March 5–9). *Genomics nursing and the EHR*. Paper presented at HIMSS18 Conference, Las Vegas, Nevada. Retrieved from http://365.himss.org/sites/himss365/files/365/handouts/550240981/handout-130.pdf

ADDITIONAL RESOURCES

Calzone, K. A., Kirk, M., Tonkin, E., Badzek, L., Benjamin, C., & Middleton, A. (2018). The global landscape of nursing and genomics. *Journal of Nursing Scholarship*, *50*(3), 249–256. doi:10.1111/jnu.12380

ClinGen. (n.d.). Home page. Retrieved from https://clinicalgenome.org

McCormick, K. A., & Calzone, K. A. (2017). Genetic and genomic competencies for nursing informatics internationally. In J. Murphy, W. Goossen, & P. Weber (Eds.), *Forecasting informatics competencies for nurses in the future of connected health*. (pp. 152–164). Amsterdam, The Netherlands: IMIA and IOS Press. doi:10.3233/978-1-61499-738-2-152

NURSING COMPETENCY RESOURCES

American Association of Colleges of Nursing. (2015). American Association of Colleges of Nursing Webinar Series: Genomics. Retrieved from https://genomicseducation.net/resource/American-Association-of-Colleges-of-Nursing-Webinar-Series-Genomics

Calzone, K., Jenkins, J., Culp, S., Caskey, S., & Badzek, L. (2014). Introducing a new competency into nursing practice. *Journal of Nursing Regulation*, *5*(1), 40–47. doi:10.1016/s2155-8256(15)30098-3

Clinical Pharmacogenomics Implementation Consortium. (2019). *CPIC® guideline for clopidogrel and CYP2C19*. Retrieved from https://cpicpgx.org/guidelines/guideline-for-clopidogrel-and-cyp2c19

Consensus Panel on Genetic/Genomic Nursing Competencies. (2009). *Essentials of genetic and genomic nursing: Competencies, curricula guidelines, and outcome indicators* (2nd ed.). Silver Spring, MD: American Nurses Association.

Greco, K. E., Tinley, S., & Seibert, D. (2012). *Essential genetic and genomic competencies for nurses with graduate degrees*. Retrieved from https://www.genome.gov/Pages/Health/HealthCareProvidersInfo/Grad_Gen_Comp.pdf

HealthCare IT News. (2018). *Bringing the EHR into the practice of Precision Medicine and genomics*. Retrieved from http://www.healthcareitnews.com/news/bringing-ehr-practice-precision-medicine-and-genomics

Jenkins, J., Calzone, K., Caskey, S., Culp, S., Weiner, M., & Badzek, L. (2014). Methods of genomic competency integration in practice. *Journal of Nursing Scholarship*, *47*, 200–210. doi:10.1111/jnu.12131

National Human Genome Research Institute. (2019, December). *Provider genomics education resources*. Retrieved from https://www.genome.gov/For-Health-Professionals/Provider-Genomics-Education-Resources

Raman, G., Wallace, B., Chung, M., Mahoney, A., Trikalinos, T. A., & Lau, J. (2010). *Technology assessment: Update on genetic tests for non-cancer diseases/conditions: A horizon scan*. Retrieved from https://www.cms.gov/Medicare/Coverage/DeterminationProcess/downloads/id49ta2.pdf

7

The Future of Emerging Technologies and Nursing

WHENDE M. CARROLL

CHAPTER OBJECTIVES

- Discuss additional emerging technologies being developed for use in healthcare.
- Identify existing and emerging technologies used in the community setting.
- Examine how novel technologies will impact health consumerism and the sharing economy.
- Explore future nursing roles that will further the use of emerging technologies in the 21st century.

CONTENTS

INTRODUCTION

There is a strong case set throughout this text for efficacious applications of emerging technologies by nurses. With technology changing daily and the immense amount of data created every hour, the nursing industry can only speculate about what their future holds regarding the future of health information technology (IT). This chapter explores more novel technologies that are in their infancy; along with current technologies, these will further the patient–nurse connection, move care out of the hospital and clinical settings, and match healthcare consumer and society demands for independence, cost-consciousness, and convenience as seen in other industries. What will be constant is that nurses will continue to hold to the mission of providing empathetic care regardless of the technology used to deliver it. The new models of care emerging that have technology at their core for improving care and outcomes add a need for expedited transformation to keep up with the changing tide. With transformed roles and new highly specialized skills and knowledge, nurses will further use data to drive quality and safety, become linchpins in health digitalization, and act as health IT innovators to drive the future of emerging technologies to serve the Quadruple Aim.

SMART COMPUTING IN CARE SETTINGS FOR CONNECTION, SECURITY, AND PROXIMITY

Ambient Intelligence

Ambient intelligence (AmI), the emerging technology used in programs such as virtual personal assistants (VPAs), including Amazon's Alexa and Google's Assistant, refers to passive digital environments that are sensitive to the presence of people, context-aware, and adaptive to the needs and routines of each end user (Edwards, 2018). Ambient abstraction—ambient lighting, ambient sound—evokes unobtrusive yet impactful personal experience as it enhances an environment. Ambience is dependent on occurrences in the real world; using Big Data, AmI applications can expertly anticipate and proactively address needs, adapt to changing conditions, determine patterns, and make predictions and recommendations to inform enhanced decision-making (Tektonika Staff, 2017), including those in clinical settings. The valuable features of AmI systems have the potential to augment our everyday lives in many areas, one being the widespread use of this innovative technology in the healthcare domain (Acampora, Cook, Rashidi, & Vasilakos, 2013).

The beneficial capabilities of AmI embody the next wave of computing (Acampora et al., 2013), and is the core of smart hospitals. Along with smart hospitals, smart homes and smart cities use intelligent agents and pervasive, ubiquitous computing networks that perceive the state of the physical environment and residents, through human–computer interaction, using sensors and Artificial Intelligence (AI) applications, and then take actions to achieve specified goals (see Figure 7.1). During perception, sensors embedded in the hospital, home, and a community generate readings while residents and things perform their daily specified routines and functions. A computer network collects the sensor readings and stores them in a database that an intelligent agent uses to generate useful

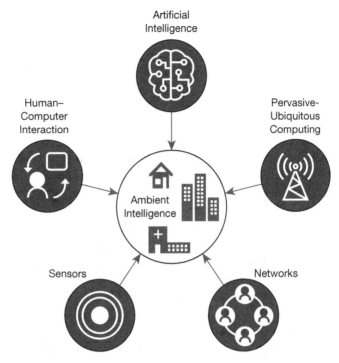

Figure 7.1 Ambient intelligence, smart homes, cities, and hospitals.

knowledge such as patterns, predictions, and trends (Cook, Crandall, Thomas, & Krishnan, 2013). Based on this information, smart hospitals, homes, and cities can select and automate actions that meet the goals of the targeted people, devices, and objects (Guo, Lu, Gao, & Cao, 2018) and provide discrete and intuitive user interfaces (Acampora et al., 2013). Smart hospitals are integral to smart homes and smart cities as patient care offered in a clinical care setting, with nurses and devices as methods of delivery, broadly impacts what happens during and after an emergency department (ED) or hospital visit or stay, and resonates into transitional care and community health. Services that assist nurses in making smarter decisions are increasingly popular because the quality of experience is increasingly essential in these applications. However, the demand for AmI services requires an extremely robust data processing capability, promoting the integration of AI in smart homes, cities, and hospitals (Guo et al., 2018).

Specific nursing applications for providing clinical care using AmI environments include completing comprehensive behavior analysis to assist living situations and using and monitoring mobile devices and wearable systems in activity recognition systems (Dey & Ashour, 2017). Also, leveraging the technology to care for people with special needs and degenerative diseases such as in the elderly, monitoring of chronic diseases, and physiological data acquisition system in ambient environments will be specific ways that nurses will interact with AmI. To exploit the AmI potential, a collective focus on all clinical technologies in the ambient environment, organizational structures, and human factors is needed by nurses (Dey & Ashour, 2017). The quest to develop, manage, and sustain smart hospitals, where digital services and tools are fully integrated into everyday patient activities, leading to better care and operational efficiency using emerging technologies such as AmI, continues. Most healthcare organizations have a vision, and continual progress is being made to solidify sufficiently smart infrastructures in coming years with countries outside of the United States currently further along in their journey (Kharbanda, Sehlstedt, Bohlin, & Treutiger, 2017).

Distributed Ledger Technology/Blockchain

Distributed ledger technology/Blockchain is one of the fastest moving and evolving emerging technologies today. As its hype is elevating, with multiple promising applications, it is a sophisticated technology that can have a significant impact on healthcare data accessibility, privacy, auditability, and efficiency. To promote better understanding and adoption of Blockchain in health IT, in 2017, the Healthcare Information and Management Systems Society (HIMSS) Blockchain Workgroup published an official definition for Blockchain. The organization classifies Blockchain as a technology for transactional applications that can be used to share a ledger, across a business network, with the ledger as the source of all transactions across the business network and shared among all participants in a secure, encrypted environment (Anderson, 2018). At the core of the technology are Blocks, or transaction records, added to the chain in a linear, chronological order where each node (a participant connected to the network) gets a copy of the Blockchain, which gets downloaded automatically upon joining (Anderson, 2018).

This technology grew out of the bitcoin technological innovation (Anderson, 2018), which was the first commercial use of Blockchain to create digital currency, or cryptocurrency, designed to ensure a trustable, decentralized, serverless, consensus-based ledger network to mitigate double-spending, forgery, and government control, authority, and third-party interference used in financial transactions (Rosic, 2018). Due to the way it stores transaction data, along with assets and information, Blockchain, as its name suggests, is just that process—blocks that are linked together to form a chain. The Blockchain expands as the number of transactions grows, and blocks record and timestamp the sequence of transactions, to verify proof of transactions that are then logged into the Blockchain, within a discrete network governed by rules agreed on by the network participants (Gupta, 2017; see Figure 7.2). Blockchain fundamentally serves as a database for recording transactions. However, its benefits—mainly immutability, or the inability to tamper with a transaction without being made too apparent—extend far beyond those of traditional databases and do not replace them. Instead, with Blockchain, data transactions, as well as asset and information records, are now shared and available to all parties participating with access to a data-based network (Gupta, 2017).

Within healthcare clinical and business processes, Blockchain can exploit its key characteristics of a ledger network. These attributes create a "trust model" for data sharing (Brodersen et al., 2016) that includes participant consensus, participants knowing where the transaction originated and how its ownership has changed over time, the inability to tamper with a transaction after recording to the ledger, and, when a transaction error occurs, using a new transaction to reverse the error. Both transactions are then visible, with a

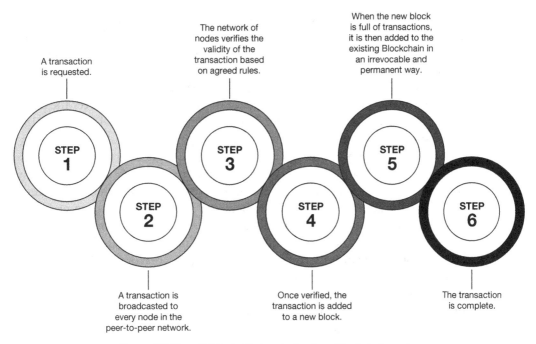

Figure 7.2 How distributed ledger technology/Blockchain works.

single, shared ledger that provides one place to go to determine the ownership of and completion of a transaction (Gupta, 2017). Currently, multiple databases store various types of sensitive patient health information in different locations, including demographics, claims, portals, pharmacies, laboratory, assessment and documentation systems, and billing. Blockchain technology can improve data exchange and interoperability to connect data sources and repositories that would allow common architectures and standards that will enable the safe transfer of personal health information among stakeholders in the network. An example would be a group of healthcare organizations united as a network where each patient care health-related event (or transaction) across the care continuum enables multidisciplinary care teams to track and update a patient's common clinical dataset each time an organization provides a health-related service (Krawiec et al., 2016).

Proposed use cases for Blockchain technology in healthcare will shape the future of clinical and administrative processes with a focus on electronic health records (EHRs), population health, telehealth, and patient payment systems. Shared assistance with medication reconciliation, patient-generated Blockchains from individual sensors and devices for sharing with patient care teams, patient and provider identity sharing, and determining insurance eligibility and processing claims, as well as identifying disease pandemics in the community, are beneficial uses of ledger technology (Gordon, Wright, & Landman, 2017). In nursing specifically, projected valuable Blockchain use cases are emerging (Anderson, 2018). In the future, ledger technology can allow nursing students to own their education through verification of educational course completion and grades, and provide a secure payment method enabling students to set up smart contracts as a method of developing and maintaining lifelong learning plans with transparency to employers to guide ongoing, meaningful professional development (Skiba, 2017). Also, nurses are able to manage their credentials independently. The development of a Blockchain infrastructure creates a global nursing credentialing platform and a gold standard of trust and portability where tokens allow a nurse to carry his or her credentials from location to location as a way for healthcare organizations to trust those credentials wherever the nurse practices, with expedited, less costly proof of licensure (Coin Review Guy, 2018). In nursing research, Blockchain ledger technology will, through immutability, reduce duplication of health science data, produce higher data quality through standardization, improve scientific tools, decrease research time from study outcomes to practice implementation, improve study completion tracking, and allow for access to more researchers and faster administrative processes including grant review and institutional review board (IRB) approval (Manion, n.d.). To further the delivery of timely and safe patient-centered care and less costly, more efficient administrative processes, the use of Blockchain ledger technology will equate to high-quality precision care, and provide nurses with the autonomous advancement, ownership, security, and ability to be purveyors of knowledge and become owners and scholars in their careers, adding value to the nursing profession.

Edge Computing

Along with understanding Big Data significance in emerging technologies, including its characteristics, sources, value, processing, and usage in various novel technologies, nurses must understand different ways to utilize data in closer proximity to healthcare settings, to ensure optimal, accurate, and expedited decision-making for patient care and administrative processes. Smart use of data occurs at the point of care delivery for nurses, and the leveraging of data processing speed regarding the immediacy of decision-making is beginning to revolutionize emerging technologies such as the Internet of Things (IoT) and AI domains. Multiple health IT vendors and healthcare organizations realize the need for real-time processing of data and usage, along with device connectivity and interoperability, in critical moments and to improve patient care and resource utilization. Edge computing meets the need for utilizing data in emerging technologies in a way that enables more reliability and timelier interventions, which is why it is a growing trend in Big Data.

Edge computing, an IT architecture aimed at resolving web congestion, moves data processing and analytics capabilities closer to the sources of data capture, making it possible to reallocate workload and computational effort, as different devices, such as IoT sensors, no longer need to send data to one central location for processing. The design distributes data to elevate bandwidth use and decreases the amount of streaming data sent to a centralized locality or the cloud for processing, enabling healthcare organizations to manage their data better (Intel, 2019a). An edge network moves the computer workload closer to the user, which reduces not only bandwidth but also latency and overhead for the centralized data center (Hamilton, 2018). Outage reduction and intermittent connectivity are also improved with edge computing because it doesn't solely rely on the cloud for processing. This architecture can aid in avoiding server down-time, ensuring reliable operations in remote locations, and avoiding unplanned downtime. With edge computing, there is also an additional layer of security as much of the data from devices don't crisscross the network but stay at the point of creation with subsequently less data in the cloud at risk for a breach or leak (Hamilton, 2018). Low latency is also a benefit as computations implemented directly on the edge devices eliminate a large network of pushing and fetching data, so the server will respond immediately once it acquires device information (Zhang et al., 2019).

Proximity-based server design enables more processing and analytics per-formance near PCs and laptops, making the use of these technologies much more ubiquitous and adds value in healthcare environments (Intel, 2019b). Deployment of servers at the edge, where data handling and analyses are closer to the source of end user data capture (see Figure 7.3), will especially advance AI program performance. Health IT leaders posit that, although AI models allow development and training to occur within the core cloud, they are more useful outside of these misty data centers, where they may lose value or become diluted. Further, utilizing edge architecture and AI can improve radiology im-aging, enhance quality outcomes, reduce errors, improve clinical diagnostics, and enable better productivity in clinical settings (Intel, 2019c). Enabling edge computing not only addresses these current challenges but also advances the future of health IT through enhancing remote monitoring, such as teleICUs, and promoting population health frameworks with patients presenting with similar conditions, some years away from experiencing the first symptom. In these scenarios, healthcare will leverage edge computing data for timely and reliable detection and treatment discoveries and preventive medicine (Bird, Strom, Schindler, Whitmarsh, & Rand, 2018).

Edge computing can support the framework for smart hospitals that, like smart homes and cities (Guo et al., 2018), allow optimal connectivity and interoperability of multiple wireless devices for people, patients, nurses, and things, such as supplies and clothing, that all together support quality patient care. Because healthcare systems are dynamic and complex systems that have unpredictable behavior, managing resources and services efficiently

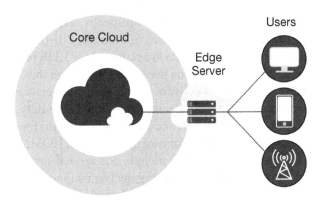

Figure 7.3 Edge computing.

is imperative today. One edge computing use case in hospital settings that can impact better use of nursing resources and increase nursing productivity is in EDs. One study by Oueida, Kotb, Aloqaily, Jararweh, and Baker (2018) used edge computing design to prove the feasibility of reducing ED wait times and patient length of stay to alleviate overcrowding and reduce the waste of resources. The researchers found that the use of edge computing with IoT to automate ED processes allowed time-sensitive storage of information in the cloud for edge server processing for fast accessibility to nurses. This technology design strategy can ensure a cost-effective, reliable computing system that integrates with medical devices for a mobile system that provides storage, updating, and immediate retrieval of electronic healthcare data by nurses to significantly improve the management of patient health records and images (Oueida et al., 2018).

EMERGING TECHNOLOGIES FOR THE COMMUNITY

The Learning Health System

The focus of novel technologies will be to work in tandem with further reaching capabilities to take on the challenges of health systems' desire to reduce costs and improve care and community-based care to improve global health. There is a call for technology and innovations to play a critical part in the continuation to develop, advance, and sustain **Learning health systems** (LHSs; Institute of Medicine [IOM], 2012). Contributing to the framework of an LHS created by the IOM in 2012 to embed quality improvement in healthcare organizations through the use of evidence-based practices and continuous improvement methodologies is the best use of data, and technological innovations are at its core for success in the high-functioning, patient-centered, adaptive care model. As described in the 2013 report, *Best Care at Lower Cost: The Path to Continuously Learning Health Care in America* (Smith, Saunders, Stuckhardt, & McGinnis, 2013), LHSs feature an underlying data-based infrastructure that enables "virtuous cycles" to improve health and lower costs based on actionable data and evidence using both patient data and biomedical knowledge generated during routine patient care. This knowledge informs care, which informs scientific evidence through the optimal use of IT and advanced data analytics (Freidman, 2014). These virtuous cycles allow nurses to learn from missteps and better leverage biomedical data and knowledge to improve care (Cummins, 2014).

Two core characteristics are required for LHS technology domain support: first, the need for real-time access to knowledge that continuously and reliably captures, curates, and delivers the best available evidence to guide, support, tailor, and improve clinical decision-making, care safety, and quality, and second, to capture the care experience on digital platforms for real-time generation and application of knowledge for care improvement (IOM, 2012b). Recommendations for the success of the LHS include accelerated integration of the best clinical insight into care decisions, using decision support tools derived from technology (i.e., AI, IoT, and EHRs), and knowledge management systems as regular features of healthcare delivery to ensure that decisions made by nurses embody current, best evidence (IOM, 2012a). The IOM also suggests digital technology developers and health product innovators create solutions to assist individuals in health and healthcare management while providing patient support within their communities (IOM, 2012b). With the essential traits and recommendations put forth by the IOM to meet the LHS objectives, healthcare organizations will welcome divergent collaborations and nurse-led innovations that encourage novel models, processes, and products to move out nations along the path toward the best care at lower costs.

Community-Focused Technology

With the imperative put forth by the IOM to support the LHS for better care and cost reduction into the community setting, the utilization of emerging technologies for public health-based conditions will drive models that support people and populations. To successfully help nurses with patient transitions of care into communities to sustain a **learning health care community (LHCC)**, where active and continuous stakeholder and community engagement aims to improve the quality and value of healthcare within a community (Mullins, Wingate, Edwards, Tofade, & Wutoh, 2018), revolutionary technological solutions that target precision public health and equity are a necessity.

This will be dependent in large part on the management of population health, defined as the health of a population as determined by health status measures and as influenced by economic, social, and physical environments, personal health practices, individual capacity and coping skills, human biology, early child development, and health services (Eng, 2004). The value-based model will improve hospital-based, transitional, and outpatient care by risk-stratifying patients, segmenting them into cohorts, and managing their conditions, diseases, and treatments to reduce costs and improve quality and care efficiency on a broader scale. Emerging technologies will enable the future development of population health programs to connect patients and providers for conditions and disease, as well as better patient engagement and overall health outcomes with the sharing of Big Data sources including those from EHR, claims, prescription history, and social determinants of health. This amassed information will work together in hardware and software solutions such as genomics, Precision Health, and predictive analytics to risk-stratify patients in the development and application of emerging technology to ensure better community outcomes.

In tandem with population health programs, healthcare organizations and health IT vendors will create revolutionary models, processes, and products to take on the most challenging population-based problems today, including serving rural health communities, increasing immunization rates, addressing behavioral healthcare, minimizing substance use disorders and self-harm, improving palliative and hospice care, and reducing maternal mortality and domestic violence (see Table 7.1). In the community setting, the next steps for current health information technologies such as EHRs, mHealth devices, and telehealth will be to extend their capabilities with the use of Big Data and emerging technologies.

Table 7.1 Community-Based Emerging Technologies

Community-Based Issue	Technologies	Novel Solutions
Rural health	IoT/Telehealth	Glooko, a companion tool for telemedicine software, enables rural health nurses to collect and synthesize diabetic patient data better remotely. Using a platform to sync diabetes monitors and other healthcare devices, nurses will better monitor patients' glucose data along with their diet, exercise, medications, and sleep patterns for more informed treatment advice and improved self-care adherence for patients with diabetes (Iafolla, n.d.)
Home health	IoT/mHealth	The tracking and trending of physiologic changes in people to detect early deterioration in the home have the potential to reduce home events and healthcare costs. A toilet seat-based cardiovascular monitoring system has been successfully demonstrated to collect blood pressure, stroke volume, and blood oxygenation accuracy consistent with gold standard measures in heart failure patients and found to reduce hospital readmissions. These types of smart systems will be uniquely positioned to capture trend data in the home that has been previously unattainable (Conn, Schwarz, & Borkholder, 2019).
Immunizations	AI/search engines	Improved influenza state-specific surveillance using autoregression algorithms with general online information (ARGONet) uses real-time data sources such as online search engines and EHR data to provide information about the present, or "nowcasting", allowing the model to enable nurses to respond to current influenza trends immediately. Together, web-based data sources with this structural network-based approach improve prediction accuracy by determining timely influenza outbreaks for more rapid intervention (Boston Children's Hospital, 2019).
Self-harm	AI/EHRs	By leveraging existing EHR data and advanced analytics modeling, it will be possible to significantly improve the prediction of death by suicide and suicide attempts over conventional self-reporting methods. Using variables including behavioral health and substance use diagnoses, emergency department and inpatient utilization, history of self-harm, and scores on a standardized depression questionnaire, these strong predictors of suicide attempt and death will help identify those at highest risk for early community nurse outreach (Simon et al., 2018).

(continued)

Table 7.1 Community-Based Emerging Technologies (*continued*)

Community-Based Issue	Technologies	Novel Solutions
Behavioral health	AI/social media	Facebook language-based prediction models can perform comparably to standard screening tools in identifying patients' depression-associated language markers—emotional, interpersonal, and cognitive—to forecast similar depression codes in the EHR in the diagnosis of depression. Using algorithms to monitor the textual content length and frequency of posts, temporal posting patterns, and demographics, **social media**-based screening methods for depression may become increasingly feasible and more accurate in the future (Eichstaedt et al., 2018).
Hospice care	AI/EHRs	Medalogix offers a novel end-of-life clinical decision support prediction solution that works in conjunction with home health agencies and hospital clinicians using predictive algorithms to consider multiple features, risk-stratify patients, and predict their decline and death within 90 days. The platform will help nurses identify hospice-appropriate patients earlier; decrease unnecessary home health utilization and frequent hospitalizations; and increase total hospice days, allowing for patients, families, and enabling nurses to begin timelier end-of-life conversations and expedite the time to receiving hospice care (Medalogix, 2019).
Opioids	IoT/smart devices	Sound Life Sciences is developing a signal processing and remote sensing app called *SecondChance* with sonar capabilities as a scalable, noninvasive, low-cost, contactless, unobtrusive method for detecting opioid overdose and connecting victims to naloxone therapy. The app runs on either a smartphone or smart speakers using frequency modulated continuous wave (FMCW) sonar, detecting high-frequency sound waves above the range of human hearing that reflect off the environment and are picked up by the device's microphones. The technology monitors a person's breathing, and when apnea is detected, it emits a loud audible alarm to summon help in the vicinity, passing the location of the person onto 911 via an application programming interface (API) from the smart device to mobilize naloxone-equipped first responders for rapid intervention (N. Mark, personal written communication, March 19, 2019).

(*continued*)

Table 7.1 Community-Based Emerging Technologies (*continued*)

Community-Based Issue	Technologies	Novel Solutions
Maternal morbidity and mortality	IoT/EHRs	An IT vendor is piloting a framework for a global system of cloud-based electronic birthing centers, where obstetrics nurses can guide skilled maternal care regardless of the mother's location. The care team will place a wearable biometric device on mothers that checks their vital signs and synchronizes them to a stand-alone EHR system via a Bluetooth device installed on computers, laptops, and tablets to pull the data directly from the wearable and transmit them to the EHR display at a nurses' station. The early warning clinical decision support system will alarm if the mothers' vitals become abnormal or drastically worsen, prompting the EHR to provide appropriate diagnosis and suggest treatment guidelines (Garage Staff, 2018).
Domestic violence	AI/EHRs	Smart machine algorithms will flag worrisome injury patterns or mismatches between patient-reported histories, and the types of fractures present on x-rays can create clinical decision support system alerts for emergency departments and clinic nurses to determine when a further assessment and an exploratory conversation regarding frequent injury is needed (Bresnick, 2019).

AI, Artificial Intelligence; EHR, electronic health record; IoT, Internet of Things.

CONSUMERISM, EXPERIENCE, AND THE SHARING ECONOMY

The Rise of Healthcare Consumerism

The baby boomer generation primarily drives healthcare costs. However, healthcare influence will shift to millennials as the U.S. Census Bureau concludes that the boomers population in 2019 will decline to 72 million and millennials will swell to 73 million (Fry, 2018). As patients, millennials will transform the future of healthcare because their use of online resources and telehealth continues to grow; they will be the first generation fully expected to share the burden of their health benefits; their beliefs that healthcare costs are too high and that third-party health payers or insurers have too much power will revolutionize care models (Vogenberg & Santilli, 2018).

Healthcare consumerism is transforming an employer's health benefit plan into one that puts economic purchasing power and decision-making into the hands of participants; supplying employees with the information and support tools needed for decisions, along with financial incentives, rewards, and other benefits that encourage personal involvement in altering health and healthcare purchasing behaviors, will make this successful (Vogenberg & Santilli, 2018). As costs for consumers continue to rise, with employers offering high-deductible health plans that shift some of the healthcare costs to employees, consumers become more engaged in getting the best value for their money and expect transparency and choice in their healthcare experience. The ability to meet consumers' needs and expectations resides with providers as they are the primary source for education, information, and the solutions that patients need to take ownership of their health providers to meet all aspects of service quality (Vogenberg & Santilli, 2018). According to Murphy (2016), successful healthcare organizations will thrive by using analytics as a core strategic foundation that includes population health, patient-care team relations, financial risk management, and consumer engagement that supports business functions and impacts the continuum care (Murphy, 2016). Nurses will be key leaders in using emerging technologies and Big Data to design and support these strategies and ride the consumerism wave of new value-based care models.

Focus on Experience

Whether it be online shopping, finding a ride across town, looking for new partners and friends, or banking, consumers are demanding convenience, affordability, security, and trustworthiness from the enabling-technology platforms that offer these services today. With more choice and increased personal out-of-pocket expenses, consumers are more selective, more cost-conscious, and look for experiences in these services that are easy, personalized, and build an emotional connection (Heath, 2017), which is furthered by emerging technologies for full engagement through their daily transactions. Consumers want an overall excellent experience at all the touch points in these services that are person-centered—this is where healthcare can learn from companies like Zulily, Lyft, Airbnb (LaBarre, 2018), Tinder, and American Express, who offer a financially appealing, premium quality of service that produces return customers.

In the case of healthcare consumers, this is steady clinical engagement, which, with consistently excellent experiences, will not only satisfy the "now economy" expectations for younger generations but will also improve their long-term health by consciously choosing, for instance, regularly accessing care for biometrics screenings and preventive visits, critical disease management, and essential prenatal and postnatal care.

To address patient experience, Arizona-based Banner Health uses technology to measure patients' experiences in real-time throughout consumers' hospital stay. The software solution, called *InMoment*, provides up-to-date information about patient needs or complaints, allowing nurses the opportunity to provocatively mitigate problems while the patient is still inside of the healthcare organization. The tool eliminates the guesswork of patient needs, using real-time data to make changes for patients on a case-by-case basis rather than using HCAHPS (Hospital Consumer Assessment of Healthcare Providers and Systems) satisfaction scores and making incremental improvements to impact quality at the point of care (Heath, 2017). Novel technologies will undoubtedly continue to play a significant role to meet the patient experience and engagement dimension of the Quadruple Aim, and the desire for shared economy services and tools for tech-savvy generations will augment interaction within the evolving healthcare system.

Furthering the Sharing Economy

Cynicism with consumerism and a desire for minimalism drives the sharing economy. Although companies are rarely the actual service provider, they act as facilitator, making a transaction possible, easy, and safe for both the provider and the user, breaking down the barriers that otherwise exist to starting a business for many people and make it both easy and lucrative to participate in a more peer-based, collaborative economy (Marr, 2016). The **sharing economy** has transformed society's overcautious behaviors from the old mind-set of don't talk to, don't get in cars with, and don't take candy from strangers. And certainly, don't let strangers in the house, to a mind-set of getting in cars with strangers, having food delivered by strangers, and inviting strangers into homes to take care of children and beloved pets, rent a room, and buy no longer wanted household items. This shift is due to convenience, affordability, and profitability, and equates to competitiveness for businesses and people. Advancing this new service paradigm is Big Data and algorithms. The once small companies such as Uber, Upwork, Thumbtack, and OfferUp would not be viable businesses on a sizable scale without leveraging a software (smart device app or website) and advanced analytics platform with the foundation of Big Data, those who have developed their platforms to allow service providers and users to connect to the benefit of both (Marr, 2016). For people to derive benefits from solutions and services offered in the sharing economy, two essential pieces are required: technology that enables scheduling of the services at the right place at the right time, and an intra-company logistics network that mobilizes that service efficiently and on time (Crampton & Reed, 2018).

What does this mean for the future of nursing and technology? Nurses will transform how patients and nurses use sharing economy services. Emerging technologies discussed in this text in conjunction with the smart apps and online platforms further mobilize more convenient, affordable, high-quality on-demand care. Increasingly, nurses will be significant players in leveraging the sharing economy in healthcare through using technology-driven peer and collaborative solutions, partnering with established sharing economy companies, and becoming nurse-led developers of innovative products, processes, and models to add value in the service ecosystem. With the demand and success of telehealth visits, tracking and trending of wearables data, and the use of smart devices for assessments and procedures, nurses will continue to revolutionize these health IT clinical services to heighten patient health engagement in more convenient locations in the community, such as the home and on the road. And, as visionaries and drivers of the future of nursing care, more nurses will be at the table as health IT executives, software product managers, chief strategists, and leaders of innovation teams as developers and providers of clinical advisory for those who develop high-value sharing economy services.

Further, nurses, along with participating in shaping the future of the sharing economy, will help to augment the positioning of third-party payers in current value-based care models. Haven, a healthcare venture established in 2019 by Amazon, Berkshire Hathaway, and JPMorgan Chase, aims to bring together the resources and capabilities of the three companies to focus on leveraging the power of data and technology to drive better incentives, a better patient experience, and a better system; as well as create better outcomes, experiences, and lower costs for their U.S. employees and families (Haven Healthcare, 2019). The company will no doubt harness the value of the sharing economy solutions they now separately offer in e-commerce, pharmaceuticals, media, real estate, food service, finance, and banking. As of the authoring of this text, no executive nursing leadership exists at Haven. On its website, havenhealthcare.com, the company is actively seeking applicants to fill clinical roles, but without specific job descriptions. This is a stark example of the immense opportunities nurses have to shape the future of a potentially game-changing healthcare provider's products, processes, and models from the ground floor.

EMERGING TECHNOLOGIES AND THE FUTURE OF NURSING

The preparation for The Future of Nursing 2020 to 2030 Consensus Study is in progress, and aims to extend the vision for the nursing profession into 2030 and steer the nursing profession to create a culture of health, reduce health disparities, and improve the health and well-being of the U.S. population in the 21st century (National Academy of Medicine [NAM], 2019). Technology will play a major part in what the committee will consider for an improved vision, and subsequent recommendations for furthering the nursing workforce and roles, research and education, and nurse well-being to serve patients throughout the care continuum focusing on health equity and disparities in communities in the next 10 years (NAM, 2019). Big Data and assistive intelligence, connected, immersive, -omics, and ledger technologies will change the face of nursing, and all have the power to significantly transform practice, education, research, and the specialty of nursing informatics (NI), requiring nurses to be diligent about being agents of change with the wave of revolutionary health IT solutions. The resounding evolution is imminent—nurses already experience it in practice—and emerging technologies will further advance the way we care, mainly how we can make decisions, improve the healthcare experience, engage and connect patients, and heighten convenience and lower cost. Today, nurses need to keep up with the pace of technology and, while remaining tech-savvy, above all, stay true to the art of healing and promoting healthy outcomes. In this age of post-humanism, as a result of technology, in what ways will nursing roles transform and how can nurses position themselves to stay relevant in this consuming wave of transformation?

High Tech and High Touch

Pressing issues in healthcare, including the changing global demographics and the simultaneous care requirements needed for dependent populations, such as the growing number of older persons worldwide (Archibald & Barnard, 2017), will influence the field of nursing and integration of new technologies to patient-centered care. Nurses' ability to balance **High Tech and High Touch**, utilizing health IT with a commitment to fundamentals of caring, for a wide-reaching impact on people throughout the care continuum, will advance the emerging technologies discussed in this text in new and exciting ways. But much is still speculative by nature of the characteristics of novel technologies, mainly their rapid growth, massive impact on society, and inherent ambiguity. Technological competency is integral to caring competency (Locsin & Purnell, 2015), yet care in the context of utilizing technology is less clear-cut, and nurses need to be anticipatory of the impacts of technology as a shared influence that humans and technologies have on the others' mutual functioning (Archibald & Barnard, 2017).

As nurses began to use emerging technologies, there has been a tendency to focus on the innovative product, process, or model instead of the person. Despite the newness and dependence on technology that can require extra time and resources and may require a skill set outside of traditional care delivery, nurses will need to keep caring at the forefront. While this is inherent with technology in a clinical setting to advocate for both patients and emerging technology, roles, attitudes, and behaviors of nurses need to change from naïve mechanized users to become more involved in technological development and delegators of how to use technology. With automation, nurses should oversee care given to patients and the coordination with other healthcare workers and technologies to ensure the appropriate delivery of patient care with technology taking care of routine tasks, and devote more time to patient interaction (Pepito & Locsin, 2018). With this, nurses can spend concentrated time getting to know more about the patient's condition and preferences, establishing an emotional connection with patients, and responding appropriately to their needs, which is key to patient experience and engagement. As technology and how nurses use it evolves, nurses should delegate which aspect of their care delivery should be technology-driven and oversee the introduction of emerging technology, ensuring their practice to be more about the universal elements of human care continuing under a novel system (Pepito & Locsin, 2018). Taking a measured High Tech and High Touch approach, nurses and patients will realize the genuine "caring" aspect.

The Fully Digitalized Nurse

As emerging technologies and automation kick in, nursing roles that will support them will evolve and intensify. For this reason, nurses should educate themselves and acclimate to advancing technology and how to supplement and enhance their skills to stay relevant in a technologically innovative future (Pepito & Locsin, 2018). Staying relevant means using novel technologies appropriately at every turn where it improves care delivery, administrative processes, the workforce, and the profession. New roles, such as nurse navigators, disease managers, care advocates, and wellness coaches brought on by the onslaught of new technology will allow nurses to change care delivery. These nontraditional roles will enable nursing to have a greater focus on spending high-value time with patients in ambulatory and community settings and population health programs, as well as embrace consumerism to connect, engage, and retain them in preventive health for long-term wellness. Committing to a transformation in roles brought on by technology will turn nurses into the stewards who fully digitalize healthcare.

One example of moving toward a fully digitalized nursing workforce is found in the United Kingdom. The National Health System (NHS) in partnership with Health Education England (HEE) and the Royal College of Nursing (RCN) has begun a movement to scale up digital literacy in society. With a focus on healthcare and technology, the 2016 RCN Congress identified an aim that by 2020, every UK nurse should be an e-nurse (RCN, 2019). This movement includes involving nursing and midwifery staff in the design and implementation of IT, increasing access to education and training, and using data to improve care (RCN, 2019). The movement also includes promoting nursing "at the forefront of new roles and models of care in a digital society" and developing "capabilities that describe . . . emerging challenges rather than competencies focusing only on current skills" in traditional roles (RCN, 2017, p. 15). This collaborative work is vital as it recognizes nurses as critical players who use technology in everyday practice to improve citizen care (RCN, 2019). In their mission, this collaboration will strengthen and transform a digitalized workforce, and equip and empower all nurses to harness and share their immense technical abilities with UK citizens. The 'e-nurse' movement is promising and is a futuristic framework and viewpoint of how to engage all nurses in technology and embrace the transformation of a workforce that is involved in the design, development, and deployment of technology in healthcare (RCN, 2019).

Nursing Informatics Advancing Emerging Technologies

While not a new specialty in the profession, **nursing informatics (NI)** will be a critical catalyst in the advancement of emerging technologies. NI is the specialty that integrates nursing and computer science with multiple information, analytical, and cognitive sciences to identify, define, manage, and communicate data, information, knowledge, and wisdom in nursing care delivery (see Figure 7.4). NI supports nurses, consumers, patients, interprofessional healthcare teams, and other key stakeholders in all roles and settings in their decision-making to achieve desired outcomes. Successful use of information structures, information processes, and IT supports the fulfillment of NI goals (American Nurses Association [ANA], 2015). Both formally trained informatics nurse specialists (INS)

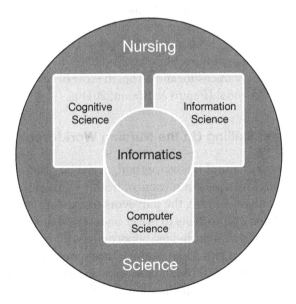

Figure 7.4 Nursing informatics framework.

and informally trained informatics nurses (IN), together known as nurse informaticists, will advance the development, adoption, and implementation of innovations that catapult nursing into the future of healthcare, furthering integrated care that improves the connection, engagement, and experience of both patients and clinicians. To that end, Siarri (2019) highlights the essential role of the nurse informaticist, and reasons that as healthcare and technology, once separate entities now fused into one daily evolving language, they have become the translators changing into health IT innovators who establish businesses, manage medical economics, create technology, and amplify the voice of end user clinicians.

With the changing tide in health IT, NI as a specialty and its roles, functional areas, and competencies will continually evolve to meet the needs of all players impacted by value-based care models. Demand for nursing education competencies in NI, and the priorities of the American Association of Colleges of Nursing (AACN), as well as the ANA, have supported the integration of these competencies into curricula and ongoing professional development for all nurses. These associations, along with leading health IT associations, including American Medical Informatics Association (AMIA) and HIMSS, also support this evolution. Interprofessional education and training will also be vital in understanding the way that technology shifts the roles of the care team (Solomon, 2019). More NIs are needed and will play a critical role in providing this education.

In the new healthcare economy and community-focused ecosystem, nurse informaticists will have a significant influence on dissolving healthcare professionals' ambivalence about embracing emerging technologies in practice. The current and future legion of nurse informaticists can be forerunners in the rapid development, adoption, and implementation of emerging technologies. For this to happen, more nurse informaticists need awareness and training to help skill up the nursing workforce and prepare for novel technologies that are changing nursing care delivery and administrative processes (Booth, 2016). NI will be the specialty that keeps nurses current and engaged with emerging technologies, including the capabilities of innovative technological advancements. As critical players on the healthcare team, they will disseminate the knowledge of how to work with these technologies, particularly those intelligent machines, and search for ways that can move these technologies to complement the task which they perform daily to ensure and dispel the fear of replacement of the human healthcare professional (Pepito & Locsin, 2018).

Nurse Scientists: Skilling Up the Nursing Workforce for Data Analytics

Nurses are natural innovators and, as the largest group of healthcare providers and therefore the largest users of health IT, the most integral human resources in the delivery of care, the purveyors of creating and sustaining the valuable relationships with patients to better understand their specific health challenges. To better understand the hidden opportunities for healthcare organizations, provider groups, payers, and patients, the future requires nurses not only to capture data but also generate, through data science, valuable data-driven insights that promote more precise, expedited, and highly reliable nurse clinical decision-making (Carroll, 2019). According to Simpson (2019), improved familiarity and comfort with Big Data analytics to scientifically use technology in nurses' work with statistics-based data manipulation for enhanced safety, quality, and outcomes will need to transpire.

To strengthen nursing education and better research, and to prove the value of nursing, nurses need to begin to strategically use big healthcare data to discover hidden patterns and trends to measure clinical and administrative performance in all settings. In the steps required to move forward with harnessing the benefits of Big Data, nurses need to learn how to use advanced programming techniques to aggregate and analyze; this is challenging, yet ultimately necessary for the profession (Simpson, 2019). There is a profound need to further train nurses at the bedside and in nonclinical settings, such as quality improvement and risk management, and improve nurses' data manipulation capabilities—not only nurse scientists trained at the doctoral level but all nurses—to advance clinical data analytics in healthcare organizations. Educating nurses in advanced programming techniques at all levels of education and various settings can help bridge this gap (Carroll, 2019).

Inherently, nursing skills are equivalent to the skills needed by nonclinical data scientists. All nurses have to manage the day-to-day patient care and ensure tasks get done in the right time frame; this requires substantial documentation and data capture with an understanding of what the data means and can transform a regular nurse role to one of a data expert (Holman, n.d.). Nurse creativity and in-depth clinical knowledge align with data scientist nontechnical skills of intellectual curiosity, effective communication, business acumen, and a strong sense of teamwork (Quora, 2017). Along with these strengths, nurses can be immensely useful in data science roles, having the innate skills of critical thinking, problem-solving, and with the strong abilities to evaluate risks and make rapid process improvements (Gutierrez, 2018).

Becoming a fully digitalized profession means technologically savvy nurses will take monumental data-driven, modern approaches to data analytics. Using data science methods, along with evidence-based care skills and abilities, a transformation of nursing roles will ensue at a critical time, where emerging technologies and workforce automation are impacting nurses. To enhance the future of care delivery and improve outcomes for patients and the community, nurses must begin to lead the charge by example to embark on a decisive mission to learn advanced data analysis, becoming the authorities as nurse data scientists and transforming nursing roles from data collectors to sophisticated data analysts to further improve the workforce (Simpson, 2019).

Nurse Innovators: The Next Tech Entrepreneurs

Nurses, more and more, are developing novel technologies, such as the emerging technologies discussed in this text, notably, healthcare moving out of the inpatient setting and into the home and community, and the rise of consumerism and the sharing economy. The Agency for Healthcare Research and Quality defines "healthcare innovation" as "the implementation of new or altered products, services, processes, systems, policies, organizational structures, or business models that aim to improve one or more domains of health care quality or reduce health care disparities" (2017, "How an Innovation is Defined").

The trend in healthcare to advance and integrate technology calls for nurses to develop creative, innovative, and entrepreneurial approaches to fill the gaps in care to address this opportunity (Darbyshire, 2014). According to Vannucci and Weinstein (2017), the current state of healthcare has led nurse entrepreneurs to focus on alternative models of care to provide patients and clients with a higher quality of life at more affordable prices and often with quicker access. Today, nurse entrepreneurs use their nursing platform to educate, empower, and engage others, with established businesses that identify existing challenges in healthcare delivery or education, develop workable solutions, and bring new products to the market (Vannucci & Weinstein, 2017).

Currently, many big technology companies have executive nursing roles at IBM, Microsoft, GE, and healthcare IT companies, including Cerner, Epic, Vocera, and CVS Health. With these high-profile roles continuing to emerge, more big IT companies will need nurse leaders who understand Big Data and innovation concepts, have strong business acumen, and possess knowledge of full life cycle product development with a mix of nursing skills such as patient and policy advocacy, health promotion, disease prevention, education, research, and consultation and advisory. Because of these autonomous functions, nurses will become the next health IT moguls who develop products, processes, and models to support the health of people and communities (Purdue University Global, 2019). Becoming executive leaders in the business of healthcare is a natural next step for the future of bringing emerging technologies to the frontline through establishing start-ups, incubators, and spinoffs, as well as brokering divergent collaborations. Because general education does not socialize nurses to administrative and leadership skills and roles in academic programs, nurses must access education to develop competencies outside of their clinical expertise. In the absence of formal education, training, or institutional support, nurse entrepreneurs typically have to build their knowledge base and best practices as entrepreneurs (Vannucci & Weinstein, 2017).

The ANA is now building a culture of innovation to help nurses develop skills that will allow for ongoing innovation, development, and implementation of emerging technologies. By collaborating with key partners, including HIMSS, the ANA uses a three-part innovation framework and innovation awards to cultivate and inspire future nurse innovators, and ignite, highlight, and celebrate nursing innovation (ANA, n.d.-a). To increase the visibility, as well as recognize and commend nurse-led innovation that improves patient safety and/or outcomes, the ANA awards nurses annually to innovate through translational research, development, prototyping, production, testing, and implementation for an innovative product, program, project, or practice transformative to patient safety and/or outcomes (ANA, n.d.-b). This opportunity advocates for and stimulates all nurse-led innovations, including the creation and use of emerging technologies, and builds nursing skills for starting businesses with health IT at its core. Nurse entrepreneurs now have opportunities and a voice with the support from nursing and health IT organizations and companies. There is also a call to nurses from other nurses who have already built health IT-based businesses to not only apply emerging technologies to optimize nursing care delivery but to take the stage in becoming health IT and innovation leaders and the cornerstones in developing emerging technologies in decades to come.

CONCLUSION

Societal and generational needs are evolving. For these reasons, optimal health literacy for all citizens with a focus on nurses to improve care using technology is essential. With the increased use of emerging technology, current and future nursing roles are and will become more transfixed on technology with the birth of more innovative technologies. The new trends of consumerism and the focus on patient engagement and experience will lead to an increase in sharable services; the face of nursing will change, and using data to provide care will advance our profession. The details about many emerging technologies in healthcare lending opportunities in the future featured in this text reflect the growing need for effective capture and use of Big Data to critically feed the technology of tomorrow. The purpose of revolutionary models, products, and processes is to assist nurses in better clinical and operational decision-making through the use of AI programs, advanced analytics such as machine and deep learning, virtual and augmented reality devices, and the IoT ecosystems to provide precision nursing care. Genomics and precision health and Blockchain capabilities will also move nurses to practice in a way that enables active use of precious healthcare data to transform care delivery and administrative processes. In the ever-evolving value-based care environment, nurses' use of novel technologies will add more value to meet the needs to impact health expenditures and provide savings and rewards for health systems and providers. A common denominator in all emerging technologies is their application for expedited, highly reliable, and efficient operations that enable the furthering of nursing knowledge for the best prognosis, treatments, and safe, quality patient outcomes. The health of people and populations, including nurses, will continue to be realized as we move further into the mid-21st century.

GLOSSARY

Ambient Intelligence: A passive digital environment that is sensitive to the presence of people, context-aware, and adaptive to the needs and routines of each end user, dependent on occurrences in the real world.

Distributed Ledger Technology/Blockchain: A technology for transactional applications that can be used to share a ledger across a business network, with the ledger as the source of all transactions across the business network and shared among all participants in a secure, encrypted environment. Transaction records (Blocks) are added to the chain in a linear, chronological order where each node (network participant) obtains a copy of the Blockchain, which gets downloaded automatically upon joining.

Edge Computing: An information technology architecture aimed at resolving web congestion that moves data processing and analytics capabilities closer to the sources of data capture, to reallocate workload and computational effort, mitigating the need to send data to one central location for processing.

Healthcare Consumerism: Transforming an employer's health benefit plans into one that puts economic purchasing power and decision-making into the hands of employees with supportive information and tools needed for decisions, and financial incentives, rewards, and multiple benefits that encourage personal involvement in altering their health.

High Tech and High Touch: Utilizing health IT with a commitment to fundamentals of caring, for a wide-reaching impact on people throughout the care continuum.

Learning Health Care Community (LHCC): Active and continuous stakeholder and community engagement aimed to improve the quality and value of public healthcare within a community using revolutionary technological solutions that target precision care in communities and health equity.

Learning Health System (LHS): Healthcare organizations that embed quality improvement, evidence-based practices, and continuous improvement methodologies into all aspects of their business model, using gold standard data analytics and technological innovations and infrastructures to leverage evidence using patient data and biomedical knowledge to inform care.

Nursing Informatics: The specialty that integrates nursing science with multiple information management and analytical and cognitive sciences to identify, define, manage, and communicate data, information, knowledge, and wisdom in nursing care delivery, supporting nurses, consumers, patients, interprofessional healthcare teams, and other key stakeholders in all roles and settings in their decision-making to achieve desired outcomes.

Sharing Economy: An ecosystem comprised of individuals, communities, companies, organizations, and associations where human and physical assets are shared among members.

Social Media: Electronic communication that creates online communities to share information, ideas, personal messages, and other content.

THOUGHT-PROVOKING QUESTIONS

1. How might the learning health system framework succeed with the use of emerging technologies in nursing practice?

2. Based on the movement of nursing care to the community, what additional public health concerns might be further assisted by emerging technology?

3. Considering current and emerging technologies in healthcare and other industries, how will health consumerism and the sharing economy grow or change value-based care models in the next decade?

4. How can new nursing knowledge skills of advanced data programming techniques and innovation solve problems in rural and disadvantaged communities?

5. Will transforming roles in nursing due to the development and adoption of novel technologies meet the need of translational research and nursing education?

REFERENCES

Acampora, G., Cook, D. J., Rashidi, P., & Vasilakos, A. V. (2013). A survey on ambient intelligence in health care. Proceedings of the IEEE. *Institute of Electrical and Electronics Engineers, 101*(12), 2470–2494. doi:10.1109/JPROC.2013.2262913

Agency for Healthcare Research and Quality. (2017). *About the AHRQ health care innovations exchange.* Retrieved from https://innovations.ahrq.gov/about-us

American Nurses Association. (2015). *Nursing informatics: Scope and standards of practice* (2nd ed.). Silver Spring, MD: Author.

American Nurses Association. (n.d.-a). *Innovation in nursing and healthcare.* Retrieved from https://www.nursingworld.org/practice-policy/innovation-in-nursing/#events

American Nurses Association. (n.d.-b). *The 2nd annual ANA innovation awards.* Retrieved from https://www.nursingworld.org/aia

Anderson, C. (2018, November). A look at blockchain and applicability to nursing. *Online Journal of Nursing Informatics, 22*(3). Retrieved from https://www.himss.org/library/look-blockchain-and-applicability-nursing

Archibald, M. M., & Barnard, A. (2017). Futurism in nursing: Technology, robotics and the fundamentals of care. *Journal of Clinical Nursing, 27*(11–12), 2473–2480. doi:10.1111/jocn.14081

Bird, B. R., Strom, D., Schindler, E., Whitmarsh, J., & Rand, D. (2018, May 16). *How emerging healthcare technology is changing the workplace for nurses.* Retrieved from https://www.hpe.com/us/en/insights/articles/how-emerging-healthcare-technology-is-changing-the-workplace-for-nurses-1805.html

Booth, R. (2016). Informatics and nursing in a post-nursing informatics world: Future directions for nurses in an automated, artificially intelligent, social-networked healthcare environment. *Nursing Leadership, 28*(4), 61–69. doi:10.12927/cjnl.2016.24563

Boston Children's Hospital. (2019, January 11). Harnessing multiple data streams and Artificial Intelligence to better predict flu: 'Nowcasting' technique enables highly accurate local flu surveillance. *ScienceDaily.* Retrieved from https://www.sciencedaily.com/releases/2019/01/190111143744.htm

Bresnick, J. (2019, April 11). Top 12 artificial intelligence innovations disrupting healthcare by 2020. *HealthITAnalytics.* Retrieved from https://healthitanalytics.com/news/top-12-artificial-intelligence-innovations-disrupting-healthcare-by-2020

Brodersen, C., Kalis, B., Leong, C., Mitchell, E., Pupo, E., & Truscott, A. (2016, August). *Blockchain: Securing a new health interoperability experience.* Retrieved from https://pdfs.semanticscholar.org/8b24/dc9cffeca8cc276d3102f8ae17467c7343b0.pdf

Carroll, W. (2019, July). Putting the 'N' in STEM. *Online Journal of Nursing Informatics, 23*(1). Retrieved from https://www.himss.org/library/putting-n-stem-call-nurse-data-scientists

Coin Review Guy. (2018, July 9). *Interview with the nurse token team.* Retrieved from https://medium.com/@CoinReviewGuy/interview-with-the-nurse-token-team-41b80714e709

Conn, N. J., Schwarz, K. Q., & Borkholder, D. A. (2019). In-home cardiovascular monitoring system for heart failure: Comparative study. *JMIR mHealth and uHealth, 7*(1), e12419. doi:10.2196/12419

Cook, D. J., Crandall, A. S., Thomas, B. L., & Krishnan, N. C. (2013). CASAS: A smart home in a box. *Computer, 46*(7), 62–69. doi: 10.1109/MC.2012.328

Crampton, J., & Reed, B. (2018, April 5). *Is the "sharing economy" the disrupter healthcare needs?* Retrieved from https://www.modernhealthcare.com/article/20180405/SPONSORED/180409955/is-the-sharing-economy-the-disrupter-healthcare-needs

Cummins, M. R. (2014). Nursing informatics and learning health system. *Computers, Informatics, Nursing, 32*(10), 471–474. doi:10.1097/CIN.0000000000000109

Darbyshire, P. (2014). An idea whose time has come: Nursing entrepreneurialism. *Whitireai Nursing and Health Journal, 21,* 9–14.

Dey, N., & Ashour, A. (2017). Ambient intelligence in healthcare: A state-of-the-art. *Global Journal of Computer Science and Technology, 17*(3). Retrieved from https://computerresearch.org/index.php/computer/article/view/1597

Eichstaedt, J. C., Smith, R. J., Merchant, R. M., Ungar, L. H., Crutchley, P., Preotiuc-Pietro, D., … Schwartz, H. A. (2018). Facebook language predicts depression in medical records. *Proceedings of the National Academy of Sciences of the United States of America, 115*(44), 11203–11208. doi:10.1073/pnas.1802331115

Eng, T. R. (2004). Population health technologies: Emerging innovations for the health of the public. *American Journal of Preventive Medicine, 26*(3), 237–242. doi:10.1016/j.amepre.2003.12.004

Friedman, C. (2014). *Informatics for the nationwide learning health system. Learning health system seminar series*. Salt Lake City, UT: Intermountain Healthcare.

Fry, R. (2018, March 1). *Millennials projected to overtake Baby Boomers as America's largest generation*. Retrieved from https://www.pewresearch.org/fact-tank/2018/03/01/millennials-overtake-baby-boomers

Garage Staff. (2018, November 20). *Using technology to fight maternal mortality worldwide*. Retrieved from https://garage.ext.hp.com/us/en/impact/hp-wonder-project-maternal-mortality.html

Gordon, W., Wright, A., & Landman, A. (2017, February 9). Blockchain in health care: Decoding the hype. *New England Journal of Medicine Catalyst*. Retrieved from http://catalyst.nejm.org/decoding-blockchain-technology-health

Guo, K., Lu, Y., Gao, H., & Cao, R. (2018). Artificial Intelligence-based semantic Internet of Things in a user-centric smart city. *Sensors, 18*(5), 1341. doi:10.3390/s18051341

Gupta, M. (2017). *Blockchain for dummies* (IBM limited edition). Hoboken, NJ: John Wiley & Sons., Inc.

Gutierrez, D. (2018). *Top jobs that pave the way for becoming a data scientist*. Retrieved from https://opendatascience.com/top-jobs-that-pave-the-way-for-becoming-a-data-scientist

Hamilton, E. (2018, December 31). *What is edge computing: The network edge explained*. Retrieved from https://www.cloudwards.net/what-is-edge-computing

Haven Healthcare. (2019). *Vision*. Retrieved from https://www.havenhealthcare.com/vision

Healthcare Information and Management Systems Society. (2017). *HIMSS Dictionary of health information technology terms, acronyms, and organizations* (4th ed.). Boca Raton, FL: Taylor & Francis.

Heath, S. (2017, March 1). *Retail consumer experience key in consumer-driven healthcare*. Retrieved from https://patientengagementhit.com/news/retail-consumer-experience-key-in-consumer-driven-healthcare

Holman, T. (n.d.). *How a healthcare data scientist can aid in value-based care*. Retrieved from https://searchhealthit.techtarget.com/feature/How-a-health care-data-scientist-can-aid-in-value-based-care

Iafolla, T. (n.d.). *3 Innovative rural healthcare tech tools*. Retrieved from https://blog.evisit.com/3-innovative-rural-healthcare-tech-tools

Institute of Medicine.. (2012a, September). *Recommendations: Best care at lower cost–the path to continuously learning health care in America*. Retrieved from http://www.nationalacademies.org/hmd/~/media/Files/Report%20Files/2012/Best-Care/Best%20Care%20at%20Lower%20Cost_Recs.pdf

Institute of Medicine. (2012b, September). *Report brief: Best care at lower cost–the path to continuously learning health care in America*. Retrieved from http://nationalacademies.org/hmd/~/media/Files/Report%20Files/2012/Best-Care/BestCareReportBrief.pdf

Intel. (2019a, January 29). Executive summary 1—From confusion to clarity: The case for edge computing. *HIMSS Media*. Retrieved from https://www.himsslearn.org/executive-summary-1-confusion-clarity-case-edge-computing

Intel. (2019b, January 29). Executive summary 2—Edge computing: Strategic considerations and benefits. *HIMSS Media*. Retrieved from https://www.himsslearn.org/executive-summary-2-edge-computing-strategic-considerations-and-benefits

Intel. (2019c, February 8). Executive summary 4—Edge computing: A sweet spot for artificial intelligence. *HIMSS Media*. Retrieved from https://www.himsslearn.org/executive-summary-4-edge-computing-sweet-spot-artificial-intelligence

Kharbanda, V., Sehlstedt, U., Bohlin, N., & Treutiger, J. (2017). *Building the smart hospital agenda: A comprehensive approach for hospitals executives to develop their smart hospital strategy and implementation program* [Whitepaper]. Retrieved from http://www.adlittle.com/sites/default/files/viewpoints/ADL_Smart%20Hospital.pdf

Krawiec, R., Barr, D., Killmeyer, K., Filipova, M., Nesbit, A., Israel, A., ... Tsai, L. (2016). *Blockchain: Opportunities for health care.* Retrieved from https://www.healthit.gov/sites/default/files/4-37-hhs_blockchain_challenge_deloitte_consulting_llp.pdf

LaBarre, S. (2018, October 9). *What the healthcare industry could learn from Lyft and Airbnb.* Retrieved from https://www.fastcompany.com/90243420/what-the-healthcare-industry-could-learn-from-lyft-and-airbnb

Locsin, R., & Purnell, M. (2015). Advancing the theory of technological competency as caring in nursing: The Universal Technological Domain. *International Journal for Human Caring, 19,* 50–54. doi:10.20467/1091-5710-19.2.50

Manion, S. (n.d.). *Distributed science value and opportunity* [Slide Set]. Retrieved from https://img1.wsimg.com/blobby/go/63238567-29f6-4c63-b86e-61d521f2d11f/downloads/1d1tfrql9_16553.pdf

Marr, B. (2016, October 21). The sharing economy—What it is, examples, and how big data, platforms and algorithms fuel it. *Forbes Magazine.* Retrieved from https://www.forbes.com/sites/bernardmarr/2016/10/21/the-sharing-economy-what-it-is-examples-and-how-big-data-platforms-and-algorithms-fuel

Medalogix. (2019). *Medalogix bridge.* Retrieved from https://medalogix.com/bridge

Mullins, C. D., Wingate, L. T., Edwards, H. A., Tofade, T., & Wutoh, A. (2018). Transitioning from learning healthcare systems to learning health care communities. *Journal of Comparative Effectiveness Research, 7*(6), 603–614. doi:10.2217/cer-2017-0105

Murphy, J. (2016). *Harnessing population health management to promote quality improvement in healthcare.* Retrieved from https://s3.amazonaws.com/rdcms-himss/files/production/public/ChapterContent/socal/HITCON16_Judy_Murphy.pdf

National Academy of Medicine. (2019). *The future of nursing 2020-2030—A consensus study from the National Academy of Medicine.* Retrieved from https://nam.edu/publications/the-future-of-nursing-2020-2030

Oueida, S., Kotb, Y., Aloqaily, M., Jararweh, Y., & Baker, T. (2018). An edge computing based smart healthcare framework for resource management. *Sensors, 18*(12), 4307. doi:10.3390/s18124307

Pepito, J. A., & Locsin, R. (2018). Can nurses remain relevant in a technologically advanced future? *International Journal of Nursing Sciences, 1*(6), 106–110. doi:10.1016/j.ijnss.2018.09.013

Purdue University Global. (2019). *Top 10 nursing trends for 2020.* Retrieved from https://www.purdueglobal.edu/blog/nursing/top-10-nursing-trends/

Quora. (2017, June 15). What are the top five skills data scientists need? *Forbes Magazine.* Retrieved from https://www.forbes.com/sites/quora/2017/06/15/what-are-the-top-five-skills-data-scientists-need

Rosic, A. (2018, September 13). *Learn what is cryptocurrency: [Everything you must need to know!].* Retrieved from https://blockgeeks.com/guides/what-is-cryptocurrency

Royal College of Nursing. (2017). *Improving digital literacy.* Retrieved from https://www.rcn.org.uk/-/media/royal-college-of-nursing/documents/clinical-topics/improving-digital-literacy.pdf

Royal College of Nursing. (2019). *Every nurse an e-nurse—Digital capabilities for 21st century nursing.* Retrieved from https://www.rcn.org.uk/clinical-topics/ehealth/every-nurse-an-e-nurse

Siarri, D. (2019, July 3). *What is nursing informatics?* Retrieved from https://www.himss.org/news/what-nursing-informatics?utm_source=twitter&utm_medium=social&utm_campaign=nurses_week&hootPostID=17708e4f014433903342d2b003764ba4

Simon, G. E., Johnson, E., Lawrence, J. M., Rossom, R. C., Ahmedani, B., Lynch, F. L., ... Shortreed, S. M. (2018). Predicting suicide attempts and suicide deaths following outpatient visits using electronic health records. *American Journal of Psychiatry, 175*(10), 951–960. doi:10.1176/appi.ajp.2018.17101167

Simpson, R. (2019, April). *General keynote address–kaleidoscope: Twists and turns in big data. Session 201*, American Nursing Informatics Association 2019 Conference, Las Vegas, Nevada.

Skiba, D. J. (Ed). (2017). The potential of blockchain in education and health care. *Nursing Education Perspectives, 4*(38), 220–221. doi:10.1097/01.NEP.0000000000000190

Smith, M., Saunders, R., Stuckhardt, L., & McGinnis, J. M. (Eds.). (2013). *Best care at lower cost: The path to continuously learning health care in America*. Washington, DC: National Academies Press.

Solomon, C. (2019, May 8). *Technology and the future of nursing—A virtual panel*. Retrieved from https://medium.com/@cassiesolomon/technology-and-the-future -of-nursing-a-virtual-panel-1981bc3a1ef0

Tektonika Staff. (2017, October 18). *What the heck is ambient tech?* Retrieved from https:// www.tektonikamag.com/index.php/2017/10/18/what-the-heck-is-ambient-tech

Vannucci, M. J., & Weinstein, S. M. (2017). The nurse entrepreneur: Empowerment needs, challenges, and self-care practices. *Nursing: Research and Reviews, 7*, 57–66. doi:10.2147/NRR.S98407

Vogenberg, F. R., & Santilli, J. (2018). Healthcare trends for 2018. *American Health and Drug Benefits, 11*(1), 48–54. Retrieved from https://www.ncbi.nlm.nih.gov/pmc/ articles/PMC5902765

Zhang, H., Zhang, Z., Zhang, L., Yang, Y., Kang, Q., & Sun, D. (2019). Object tracking for a smart city using IoT and edge computing. *Sensors, 19*(9), 1987. doi:10.3390/ s19091987

Index